Detox After Covid and Thrive

Detox After Covid and Thrive

ISBN: 978-1-923122-40-6 (paperback)

Published in Australia by Wendy Daniel.
Printed in Australia by InHouse Publishing, Print & Design.

IN HOUSE PTY LTD PUBLISHING

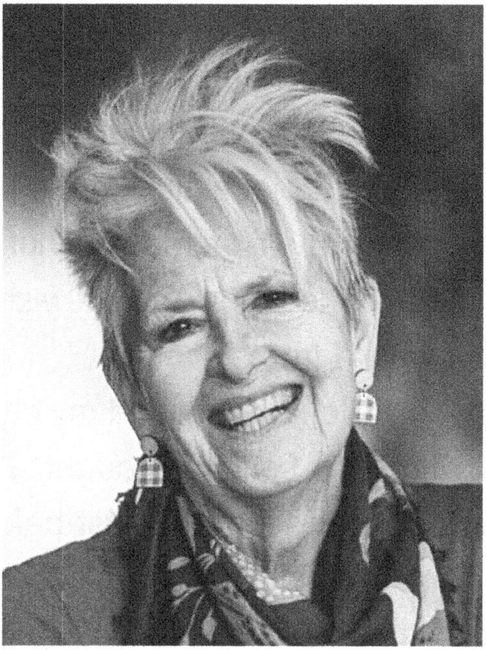

Wendy Daniel

Dear Readers

Who am I and how do I come to be putting together a book like this? I don't have a medical background which is a big advantage. I can write as I see fit without risking my career and my income as your local doctor, nurse, naturopath or midwife would. Unfortunately, these people are bound by very strict guidelines as to what they are allowed to tell us. These guidelines are instilled during their training and strongly reinforced by censorship, their own unions and their need to earn a living. Sadly, these rules are not always in place for our benefit, but to maintain pharmaceutical profit and control. This is an opinion ever increasing numbers of us have reached over decades and we wish with all our hearts that it wasn't true.

Like most people, I vaccinated my children many years ago without a second thought. I believed in vaccines without question until just before the birth of my first grandchild in 2009 when I decided to learn more. I was puzzled to find only the vaguest of vague leaflets at the doctor's office and soon chanced upon many detailed studies, facts, and courageous voices proving to me that vaccines were far from safe or effective.

If you're not yet aware of this, you can blame the vast amount of censorship which has always surrounded the vaccine issue from its earliest days. If you are interested in more information on this, you might like to read my book **Vaccines, Myths and Facts**, now in its 4th edition. You can check out the website links at the back of the book. I've been studying the vaccine issue as a lay person ever since.

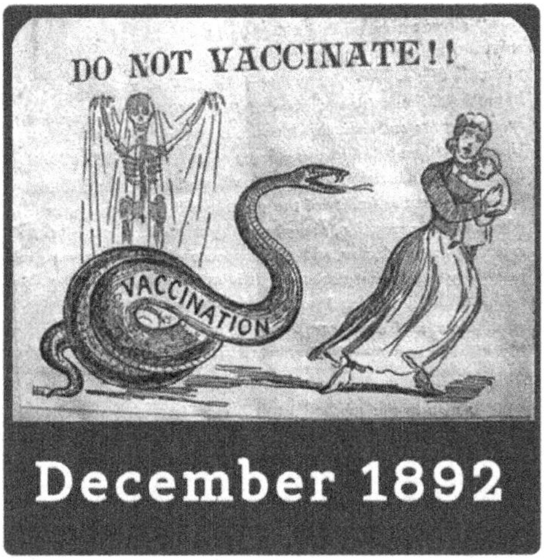

Governments around the world have been hiding this evidence for years.

If you know where to look, the scientific proof that vaccines routinely cause harm, suffering and even death has grown to avalanche proportions and now includes independently funded real life studies, testimony under oath from the pinnacles of the industry, and powerful health department documents. The evidence is clear. I no longer believe that vaccines have actually helped humanity at all.

When covid came along, the whole situation blew up in a big way. Coronavirus (common cold) vaccines had never even made it successfully through studies on animals, let alone humans. We knew that the injections were wildly experimental and completely different from anything we had seen before.

Those of us who were concerned about how this might turn out were silenced as usual. We were turned away from our favourite shops, cafes, restaurants, family gatherings and even our own workplaces like lepers in a wave of discrimination we had never known before.

Our warnings and tried and tested remedies were ignored and, horrified, we had to watch the injection roll-out from the side-lines. If you're suffering, or believe you might be suffering from covid or the injections, you're not alone. Mainstream media is still attempting to cover up the numbers, but there are many hundreds of thousands of people around the world in this situation.

This book isn't about politics, human rights or betrayal. These conversations are vital, but need not concern you at this stage. It's about how you can maintain and regain your health after covid and its treatments.

Even now in 2024, it's still early days in a brand new and very complex situation, but help is available.

This book will:

- give you some simple things you can do yourself to detox and build up your health.
- show you when you need a practitioner.
- show you how to find a good one.
- list supplements, treatment protocols and tests you might ask your practitioner about.
- point you in the direction of independent medical studies at the leading edge of covid treatment research, in Australia and around the world.
- give you some successful case histories of recovery after covid shots.
- show your practitioners some solutions they may not have considered.
- give you real hope for the future.

I am joined on this mission by a great friend and naturopath, Lee Clarke. I'm so grateful for her help and oversight with this so together we can give you some clear, simple, safe advice, guidance and encouragement.

I am also deeply grateful for the naturopaths who shared their successful case histories, Lee Clarke, Patricia Vandenberg-Smith, Rebel Tucker and a fourth professional who wished to remain anonymous. These solutions are working.

If you have lingering effects from covid infection; if you feel that your health has worsened since getting covid injections, or even if you just feel the need to detox from the crazy polluted world we live in, you're in the right place. This book is for you.

Whatever your circumstances, we hope you will find it useful to educate yourself and take full responsibility for your own health into the future.

Love and light,

Courage and strength

Wendy Daniel

March 2024

My website is: *https://www.lightoftruths.net/*

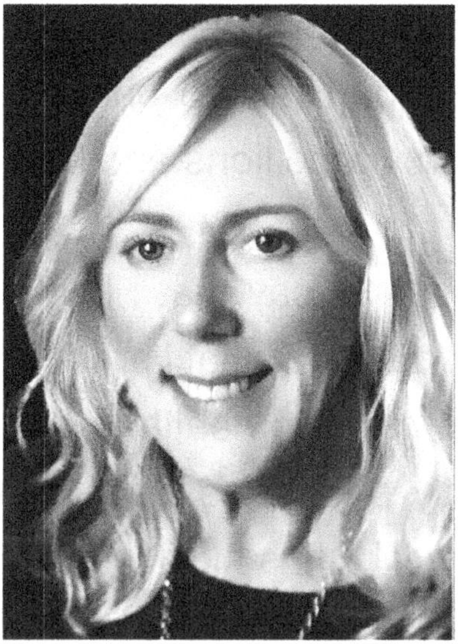

Lee Clarke - Naturopath

N.D Dip.Irid Dip.Mech Cert Hom

My name is Lee Clarke and I have been a qualified Naturopath for 26 years.

Along my journey I have added qualifications in massage, yoga, and fitness which has seen me working in a broad range of health and fitness arenas including running a clinic specialising in women's hormonal health, as resident naturopath at a holistic drug and alcohol rehabilitation centre and assistant manager, head nutritionist and fitness coach at a boutique health and fitness centre.

Each and every one of these experiences added to my level of expertise and understanding of the body and different conditions and how to treat them successfully.

It would be fair to say that I love natural health and fitness and practice what I preach with a lifetime of dedication to my own health and fitness regime. I can confidently say it has carried me through to where I am now which is high energy and strong in body mind and spirit.

I focus my attention on helping people to heal their physical bodies as I believe the body is the home for the mind and the spirit and a strong vibrant body can be the gateway that allows your soul to soar.

In the last three years in particular I have swung my attention into helping people to recover from multiple bouts of the illness of covid or covid vaccine injuries, which have left them with chronic, random and debilitating symptoms which are often dismissed by their own doctors.

I have dedicated many long hours into researching, listening and collaborating with many great doctors, scientists and natural therapists from around the world who fortunately have come up with some treatments that are working. The huge blessing is they are natural products and I have now successfully helped people to recover to full health using these methods

Lee Clarke

April 2024

My website is *www.thebodyofnaturalhealth.com.au*

The information in this book is shared in good faith to help you recover.

We're putting in a disclaimer here that we take **NO** responsibility for any of it, or what you do with it. It is (as they say) for entertainment purposes only.

You and only you are responsible for your own or your child's body, and this might be one of the most important lessons of all in the post covid era.

I think of this book like a lifebelt that someone in a rowing boat might throw to a swimmer out at sea.

This is the best we can do ... throw you a lifebelt and point you in the direction of the shore ...

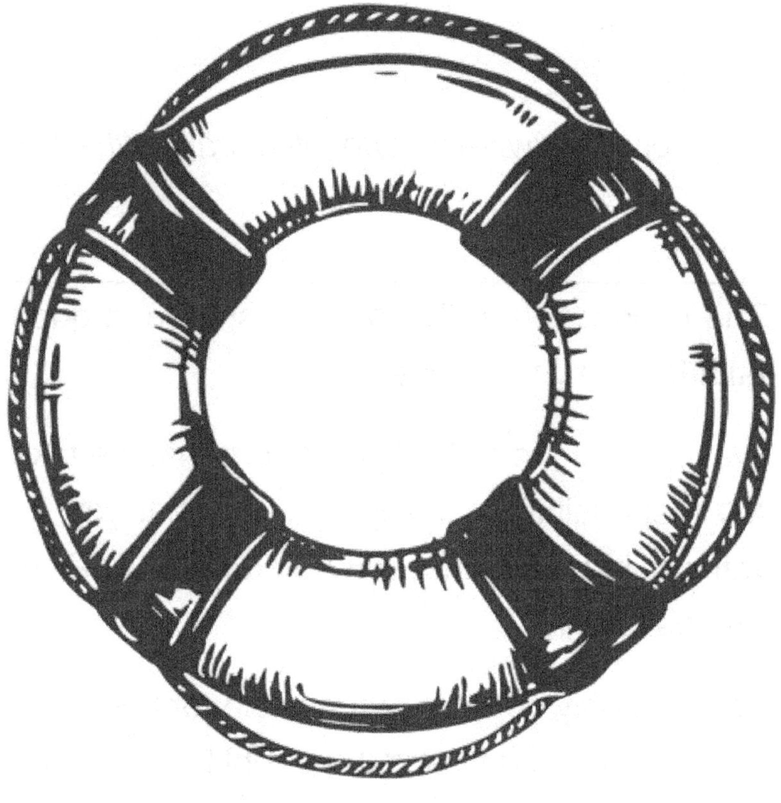

Your Life in Your Hands

Sometimes we're cruising through life and it suddenly takes a turn and we find ourselves on the open sea without a paddle, or even a compass. We have no idea which direction to take to find the shore. We didn't know what we didn't know. We find ourselves in unchartered territory without the knowledge of where to turn or even who we can trust to point us in the right direction. You may have trusted your family doctor, the local hospital, your employer or the news media.

Now may be a good time to reconsider this blind trust and become your own expert to participate actively in your own healing.

So far, many of the experimental injections being given appear to be saline and harmless. I hold the faith that this is true. I hope with all my heart that we and all our families are among the lucky ones. The sad fact is that in 2024, death rates are still approximately 15% higher than in the pre-covid injection era.

Dr Peter McCullough is one of the most published and respected doctors of our time and has been a courageous and outspoken voice in the post covid era, quoting robust published data in all his statements. He points out that approximately 30% of people who took the shots apparently have no symptoms at all. It's as if they never got a shot. Just over 60% have a few apparently minor issues but 4.2% have major issues. In early 2024, most of us know of someone who has 'died suddenly'. Many people have noticed significant health challenges after taking the shots or being intimate or even close to someone who had, especially in the few days and weeks after injection.

At this stage in early 2024, studies appear to show two main damaging ingredients in the shots, spike proteins and lipid nanoparticles. There may well be more, but we'll focus on those for now in the hope that in removing these unwanted proteins, the body is more able to clear any other nasties, cancers, parasites or heavy metals that might be causing issues.

Spike proteins from the injections appear to multiply in the body as it struggles to get rid of them. We might think of them like glass splinters or microscopic versions of those scratchy little seeds you get in your socks when you walk in a field. They're very irritating and if there's a lot of them and they're in there for a few hours your skin will be sore and inflamed when you finally pull them out.

Lipids are fats and lipid nanoparticles might be thought of as these sharp little seeds dipped in oil so they slide even deeper down into your sock and cause even more damage and irritation. If they find their way to the heart they can result in myocarditis, which is inflammation of the heart and pericarditis which is inflammation of the outside layer of the heart. Other organs are also vulnerable.

We everyday people had never heard of these conditions before because they used to be issues that heart specialists might see a handful of times in a whole career. Since the covid shots rolled out, they see them every week, often in young people. Other organs, such as the brain or the reproductive organs can also be damaged by inflammation from the shots. The immune system is sometimes disarmed so cancers can be triggered and accelerated as turbo cancers. Sometimes the symptoms are so unusual and diverse in a single patient that conventional medical diagnosis and treatment becomes difficult and people can be told (annoyingly) that, 'It's all in your head.'

OpenDAEN.Info

There have been nearly 140,000 adverse event reports for covid injections in Australia. Thanks to the work of a group of dedicated volunteers, the OpenDAEN.info website was launched in January 2024. This website shows the covid shot adverse reaction information gathered in the government Database of Adverse Event Notifications. The difference is that (unlike the government site) it displays the information in a format that is transparent, easy to read and understand. On this site, they show you how to lodge an adverse reaction, and you can even see injection batch numbers linked to reported injuries and can check the profile of the batch numbers you received.

As at early 2024, there's no way of knowing exactly what was in the individual shots you were given. They were all experimental, the batches varied wildly and vaccine reactions are random and vary greatly with each individual.

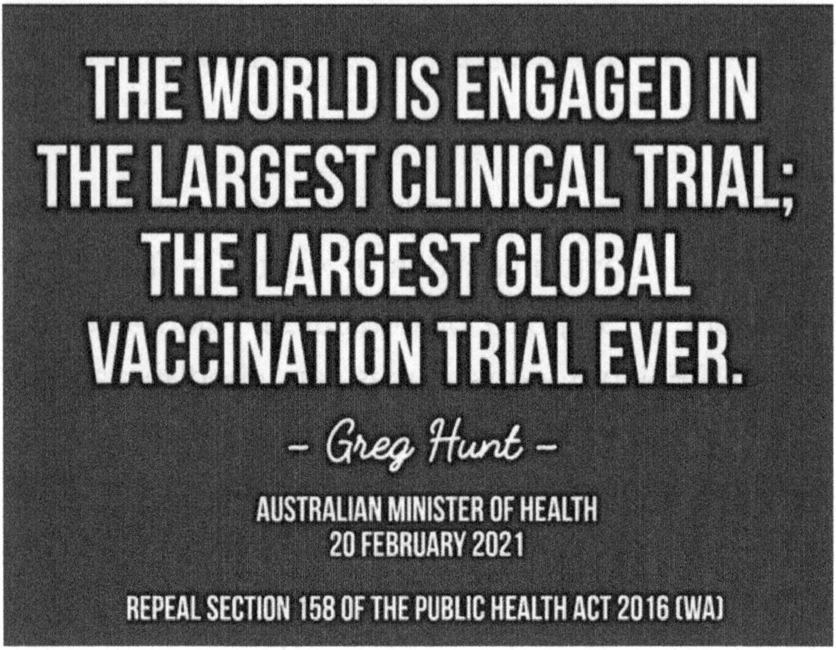

Greg Hunt tells the Australian public they are engaged in a trial - February 2021
https://fb.watch/nq4Vv77cTU/?mibextid=v7YzmG

Even if you haven't taken a shot, environmental toxins, shedding, parasites, moulds, bacteria, pesticides, and other nasties in foods, medicines, injections, vaccines, water, soil and air may have taken their toll without you being aware of it.

What can you do?

The answer is in your own hands. The time for obediently taking pills because your doctor says so is over. The real, safe, tried and true covid prevention and early treatments the industry **did** have in the early days of 2020 could easily have been packaged up into handy kits with relevant vitamins and minerals and made available at the local pharmacy or doctor's office. **This would have avoided the whole covid saga.**

There is an old truism, 'A stitch in time, saves nine.' It comes from a time when more of us mended our clothes rather than throwing them away. It works in health as much as it does in life generally. Let's use the car analogy. Most of us know that if our car starts making odd noises or the dashboard starts flashing with orange lights, we need to take it to the nearest garage as soon as possible. We know we have to get it fixed before it gets worse and the engine blows up.

Hydroxychloroquine and Ivermectin were both found to be highly effective in the early treatment of covid. They were no longer protected by pharmaceutical industry patents keeping their prices up and were being widely produced around the world for a few cents a packet. Both had been used safely in millions of doses for over 40 years. Vitamin D, C and zinc were vital in protecting the body and were also ignored in the mainstream. These simple early solutions were tossed aside, demonised and banned while people were told to wait at home until they couldn't breathe before coming in to hospital for help. This is like putting off taking your car to the mechanic until smoke is billowing from the engine.

Rushing to hospital for emergency Remdesivir and ventilator treatments proved to be expensive, dangerous and deadly.

> If you were to design a perfect drug for the treatment of covid, it would be Ivermectin.'
>
> *Paul Marik, world renowned critical care doctor and founding member of the Front Line Covid Critical Care Alliance*

'There are now 100 studies that show that Ivermectin had profound benefits. Generally speaking, a 70% to 85% reduction in hospitalizations and deaths. It was really a miracle drug.'
Robert F Kennedy Jr

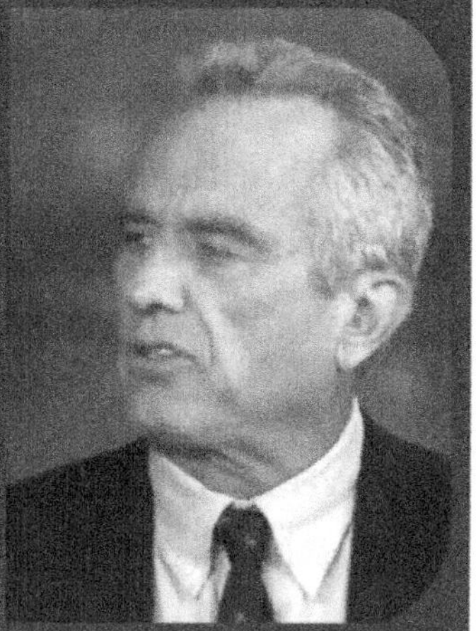

Thankfully, there are now many groups of ethical doctors around the world who are doing their best to find real solutions for you. A few are listed later in the book. In these fast-moving times, this pioneering work is every bit as important to your doctor and your naturopath as it is to you.

In essence, all illness is caused by having a body so toxic that the cells can no longer cope, being deficient in a nutrient or being out of balance with too much of a nutrient. As a general principle you need to detox and build up a reserve of essential nutrients so your body recovers its strength and resilience. With that foundation, you'll be fit and strong enough to take advantage of specific treatments targeted towards your specific recovery needs as they come along.

I've collected as many starter points as I can for this line up and I believe many more solutions will come to light as time goes by. There are things you can and should do for yourself, and there are more specialised treatments where you'll need a guiding hand.

I was once a personal trainer and realised a simple basic principle. I learned that if someone was in good health and just wanted to lose a couple of kilos and improve on their existing fitness, they didn't really need much one-on-one personal help. They could come in to the gym, do a few classes, clean up their diet a bit, and they'd reach their goals pretty quickly without too much problem.

If you haven't had the covid shots and are in good health you might be in this category. You can check out the starter points here, maybe add a couple to your normal health routine, and you'll be fine.

If someone came into the gym with an injury, a big goal, a lot of extra weight or a chronic condition, then expert guidance and encouragement along the way was vital. These people didn't necessarily have a quick or easy journey ahead of them. Time, persistence, discipline and faith in themselves and their mentors were essential.

If you've taken the covid shots or have other health issues, you may be in this category. You may need to find a trusted naturopath or, very aware, open-minded doctor to guide you through. (Sadly, there aren't too many of these doctors around).

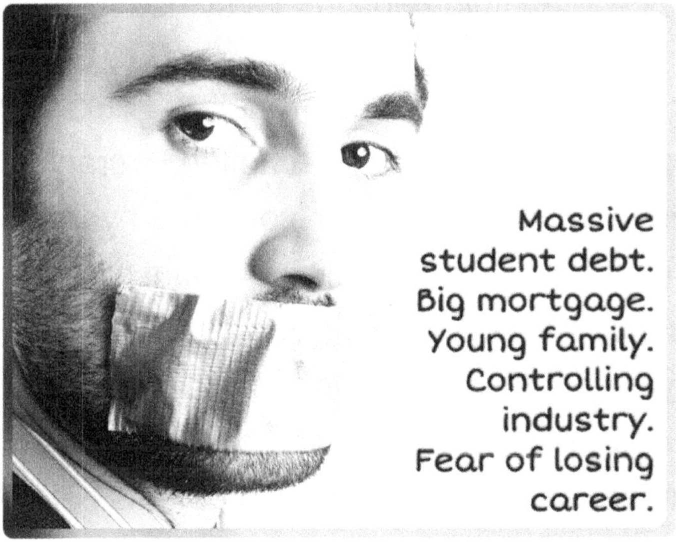

Conventional western medicine is great in an emergency or to set a broken bone, but as a whole it tends to prefer labelling and covering up symptoms rather than getting to the heart of the issue and helping the body to heal itself. The doctor's office may be handy for blood and other testing but, unless he's had a big change of heart, the medical practitioner who injected such highly experimental and untested toxins into your body without your informed consent, may not have any real solutions for you.

> If you've had the shots, I believe it's wise to be extra cautious and seek independent health advice even if you don't have symptoms.

Treatments like naturopathy, homeopathy, chiropractic, massage, nutrition, cranio-sacral therapy, physiotherapy, colonic hydrotherapy, acupuncture, reiki, wholistic counselling, yoga, frequency and energy work, and a host of others work with your body so it can heal itself. In everyday life, if you nurture your health and don't poison yourself too much, you can avoid most problems before they even come up. Going back to our car analogy, it's like keeping our vehicle serviced and and doing regular checks of tyres, oil and water levels.

'First do no harm', once thought to be the guiding principle of doctors, is taken very seriously by these professionals.

Your magnificent body

Let's take a moment to wonder at the magnificence of your body. It's made up of approximately 30 trillion cells, all working in harmony to preserve the temple of your soul. You can work on your computer, listen to music, talk on the 'phone, breathe and tap your feet while your food is digested and waste material is stored until you're ready to get rid of it. Your heart beats steadily in the background pumping your lifeblood around 10,000 kilometres of cardio-vascular system at the rate of about five litres (quarts) a minute. The lymphatic system holds a similar amount of fluid but without a pump, so it depends on your activity to work properly.

A perfect baby grows from just a couple of tiny cells and we now know that a mother's milk adapts its nutrition to meet her baby's ever changing daily needs. Annoying symptoms are often signs of your body trying to rid itself of toxins and keep its balance. Given the right resources, your body's capacity to heal itself is immense.

Some simple things you can do yourself to support your health after the experimental shots

Part of this journey is to really think about what you're doing, where your food comes from, and what it does to your body.

I first started to wake up to this in my late twenties when I was working on some brochures for a small farm animal feed company in North Yorkshire. This tiny company had a full time, fully qualified animal nutritionist who patiently spent hours with me, trying to explain the various nutrients in the feed products while I struggled to grasp both what he was talking about and how much the farmers might understand of it. (Healthy birds and animals are crucial to farmers.) Somewhere in this process, I started to wonder what on earth we were eating? It was something I'd never thought about before. This isn't too bad if, like me, you ate sensibly in childhood and carried that on in life, but you may not have been so lucky. We are what we eat and some of you may have woken up to find out that you're made of junk food.

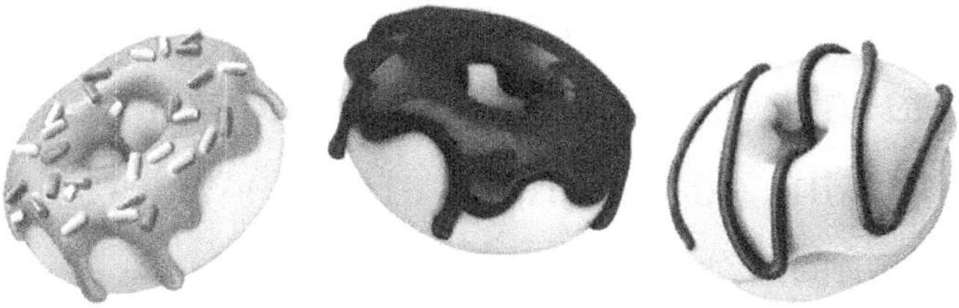

Virtually everything you read about healthy eating has the same reminders:

Eat organic and local as much as you can.

Grow your own produce or shop at farmers' markets and whole food stores rather than supermarkets for cleaner, more nutrient rich, organic produce grown by small farmers or gardeners you can trust. Vegetables, herbs and salads are your friend and many health advisers advocate a mainly plant-based diet. Salads and vegetables can be eaten raw for maximum nutrition or prepared simply in ways your great-grandmother might recognise. I think it pays to look at your individual heritage here. What would your great grandparents have eaten? This varies hugely depending on which country they lived in and it makes sense to me that what worked for their bodies, might just work for yours.

> We are of the earth and to live our best life, what we eat should be grown in good earth or have lived on the good earth or in clean waters during its lifetime.

Vegetables

Let's look in a little more detail at vegetables. Large supermarket chains are more likely to sell produce which looks good, but which may be grown hundreds of kilometres away in exhausted soils lacking in important nutrients. They may have been sprayed with poisonous chemicals to kill weeds and insect pests, and could have been stored for weeks or even months. Many suppliers do their best within this system, but big supermarkets have a near monopoly in the market and are ruthless in demanding perfect looking produce at cheap prices because that's what their customers want.

You get to choose and every dollar you spend is a vote.

If you choose your suppliers carefully at your local produce market, you'll find wonderful seasonal produce grown in real, nutrient rich soil, picked fresh that morning or at least the day before. It won't have been sprayed with anything poisonous and it usually looks as fresh as a daisy. You can even have a chat with the grower you're supporting.

It's a richer experience all round.

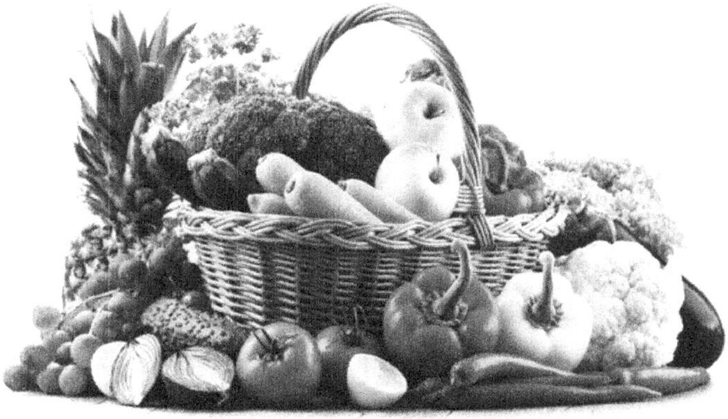

Eggs

Let's look at eggs: one carton of eggs comes from poor, caged balding chooks who've eaten the same cheap pellets all their lives and have never walked on grass, felt the rain or seen the sun. If you buy these eggs, the nutrition they give you is sadly lacking, just like the cheap pellets (complete with yellow dye to make the yolks look good.) You're also voting with your dollars and telling the egg producers, the supermarkets and the world at large that you're ok with keeping chickens indoors in cramped cages.

So they keep on doing it.

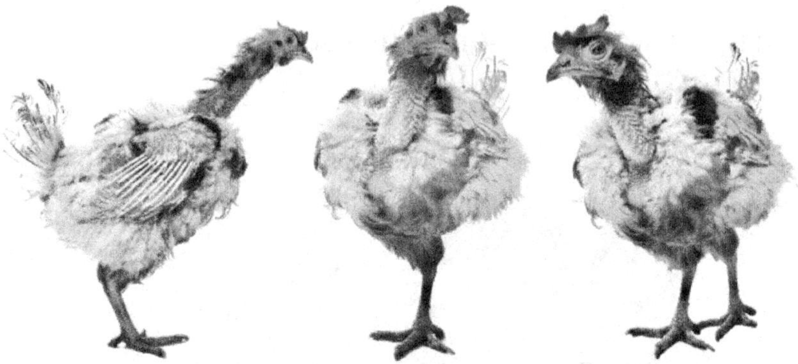

The other carton of eggs comes from happy, healthy, glossy-feathered chooks who are scratching happily around with their mates in a nice big meadow and eating a variety of nutritious bugs, worms and greens. The nutrition you get from these eggs is vastly superior. You're also voting with your dollar and telling farmers that these are the eggs you want. You're supporting these natural farmers to do the right thing. There's been a trend in this direction, but we still have a long way to go.

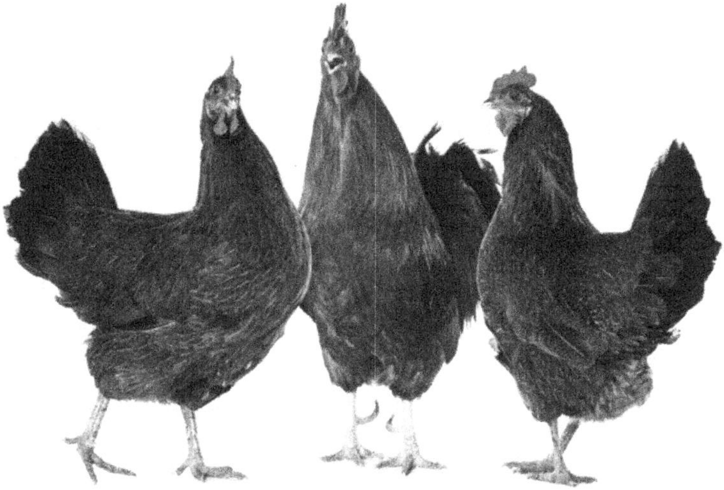

This comparison also applies to our other choices. Fatty fish, sardines, mackerel, wild caught salmon, oysters, eggs, butter, cheese, yogurt and organic, naturally raised chicken, rabbit, lamb, pork and beef offer us a wider variety of nutrients than we can get from salads and vegetables alone.

If we're going to eat these foods, it's always best to choose organic, grass fed, free range, and wholesome farming practices that keep both the soils and the animals in peak condition. This produce may cost a bit more than the factory farmed equivalent but the quality and nutritional value to you will be far better.

LESS

Avoid sugar in all forms apart from stevia. Sugar plays havoc in the body, including the brain and is apparently more addictive than cocaine. I've never had cocaine but I know I've battled sugar addiction all my life. I think I'm winning most of the time and my own strategy is simply not to have anything sugary in the house. Your family might protest but they'll all benefit massively from this policy as well.

Avoid high fructose corn syrup. Processed foods are laden with it under a variety of names. It sounds so fruity and natural, doesn't it? Sadly no. This is nearly half and half glucose and fructose. Glucose can be digested fairly easily in small quantities, while fructose can only be digested by the liver. Apparently, it's the fastest way to fatten up your liver and your waistline.

Avoid junk foods. Those **food-like products** that fill **most** of the supermarket shelves. Generally speaking, the longer the ingredient list and the more words and numbers you don't understand, the more likely it is to be full of harmful, ultra-processed and unhealthy ingredients.

Some foods are easy for us to let go of, but many of us still cling to a few of our old favourites. *It's worth spending a bit of time and energy to find or make healthy alternatives for these damaging die-hards, especially as these may be the things we eat regularly.*

Avoid Glyphosate and other herbicides and pesticides. If your food isn't **organic** or **spray free,** you can bet your bottom dollar it's sprayed with something nasty that might just be accumulating in your body, waiting to cause trouble.

Avoid legal and illegal drugs as much as possible, including paracetamol and other over-the-counter medication.

This may be easier said than done and professional help is often needed to ease off many substances gradually over weeks or months. It's worth the effort because many of them are toxic long term and hide important symptoms. There is certainly a place for minimal use of conventional medicines.

but if you're careful with nutrition, supplements, natural treatments and exercise, you don't usually need your health and wellbeing to be propped up with medication at all.

Avoid smoking. No surprises here. Vaping isn't any better. Inhaling any sort of artificial smoke, fumes or even artificial candle scents is irritating for a reason. Our lungs know what's good for them, and it's not fumes.

Avoid seed oils. Seed oils are often called vegetable oils and include canola, sunflower, soy and corn. They look so clean, clear and healthy sitting there on the shelves, but they're not. They're usually genetically modified, which means that your body struggles to even recognise, never mind process them. Instead it just stashes them away for years … presumably on your belly and hips. They increase inflammation in the brain and we're eating vastly more of them than we did just twenty years ago. We get great nutrition from organic whole seeds such as sunflower, pumpkin, and sesame but we don't find seed oils in nature because they're always tucked away safely inside these crunchy fibres.

Avoid margarine. Margarine is a highly processed non-food. That same damaging seed oil is heated, dyed yellow and processed some more to make it look like butter in its little plastic box. There are very few nutrients in this concoction so they may throw in a few to make it seem healthier. It's an impostor for an excellent food that you could make yourself and that humankind, at least in the Western world, has eaten for millennia.

Reduce wheat, bread, gluten, rice, and pasta. These simple, often highly processed carbohydrates really act as fillers for real, nutrient dense foods. Dr Paul Marik tells us that humans can easily survive without simple carbohydrates. In days gone by, foods like bread, pasta and Yorkshire pudding were often served *before* the main protein and vegetables to fill up the hungry stomachs of people who had been working in the fields all day. Mothers of lanky teenage boys with fast metabolisms and hollow legs know this strategy well, but in today's world of sedentary jobs, mineral deficiencies and expanding waistlines, most of us don't need fillers any more.

If we're not working it off immediately, many of these white carbohydrates spike our blood sugar and insulin levels even more than plain sugar and then convert it to fat on our bellies and hips. White supermarket bread is only soft and fluffy because most of its real nutrients have been removed.

If you feel you can't live without bread, organic whole grain sourdough is one of the best choices.

Reduce alcohol. It's better to think of alcohol as an occasional treat rather than a habitual crutch to help us get through our day, if we can. I know someone who was never a big drinker but who gave up his weekly tipple for months during a stressful time just in case he was tempted to use it more often to blot out reality. Alcohol is highly acidic in the body, which isn't good, and it's very expensive. (I ventured into a bottle shop in my little town on a rare visit recently and was shocked to see the vast range and glitzy packaging sparkling seductively under the lights.) If you're an occasional drinker, you might like to check out the expanding range of non-alcoholic beers, wines or cocktails and it might be an idea to seek help and support sooner rather than later if you feel you could be drinking too much.

Reduce Stress. We might need enough stress in our lives to get us off the couch, but long-term stress is damaging. It all started back in the caves when fear spiked our adrenalin so we could run away from lions, wolves and scary enemies with clubs. This response took all the energy away from our normal bodily functions like digestion and other everyday responses and directed it all into the heart, lung and muscle energy we needed to fight or escape. The problems start when we feel those ongoing stresses about losing our jobs/paying the bills/ that important meeting/driving in heavy traffic/getting to work on time etc, etc, etc. This constant stress means that those important routine body functions are neglected and the body starts to show extra signs of wear and tear.

Things to consider...

Oils

The best oils are olive, sesame or avocado oil for salads and coconut oil for cooking. Animal fats like butter and lard aren't the demons we've been led to believe either. Organic butter from grass fed cows is a valuable source of fat-soluble vitamins like Vitamin A, D, E and K2 which are needed for your body, brain, and digestive system. Our bodies make a large amount of cholesterol anyway and doctors are now questioning the whole dietary cholesterol issue, with many of the most ethical voices stating that the 'low fat' bandwagon, with its high sugar, high carbohydrate recipes, has actually been more harmful than the original, organic foods our great-grandparents used to eat.

Dr Eric Berg talks about the benefits of butter.

https://youtu.be/JttjTjKEpuc?si=RIwHC_LiYIxleaen

> Many of the things we've been taught to think of as healthy in recent years are actually based on tiny amounts of actual studies and large amounts of profit-driven marketing, so it really pays to use our common sense and think carefully about the choices that are right for us.

MORE

Clean water. Invest in a good water filter which removes fluoride. Fluoride is a known neurotoxin but isn't removed by a lot of filters (I have a Waters brand one which filters out fluoride and an impressive line-up of other toxins.) Avoid drinking water straight from the tap. It turns your kettle brown and usually tastes polluted anyway. A shower head filter or a whole house filter is a great idea if you can afford it.

Organic salads and vegetables. We're all different and if your heritage is from countries with long, cold winters, the chances are you don't turn to salads as readily as people from warmer climates where such things were available for much of the year. If your gut health is good, organic raw salads and lightly cooked vegetables, especially at the start of a meal, are a wonderful basis for a healthy life.

Celtic salt. Our bodies are crying out for high-quality nutrition: vitamins, minerals, protein and living enzymes. **Barbara O'Neill** has a wealth of common-sense health information on YouTube and recommends taking a large pinch of sea salt before every half glass of pure water. This makes a lot of sense when we remember that we are of the earth, like the water in the oceans. She explains that high quality Celtic sea salt contains **92** trace minerals in a form your body's cells can access easily and at a price you can easily afford.

Exercise. If you took the shots and have experienced any issues, check very carefully with your wholistic practitioner before doing any but the gentlest exercise. We've now seen that intense exercise after the shots can make heart issues (which you may not even be aware of) much worse.

If you haven't taken the shots, it's worth finding some exercise you like, and will do happily every day. Movement is vital. Yoga, pilates, stretching, weights, walking, running, skipping or team sports, the list is endless. The main thing is that we do it every day. Apart from all the obvious reasons, your body contains about 5 litres of lymph (that's about the same quantity as the blood.) Its job is to clean out toxins and, unlike the blood, the lymph doesn't have a pump. That's your job. When you exercise, especially on a rebounder, (a mini trampoline,) the lymph is pumped around the body and you feel tired but energised and refreshed afterwards. If you drive to work and sit around at a desk all day, (or sit on the couch writing a book about health) it's not going to take long before you feel 'sluggish'. A good word for a load of toxic lymph with nowhere to go.

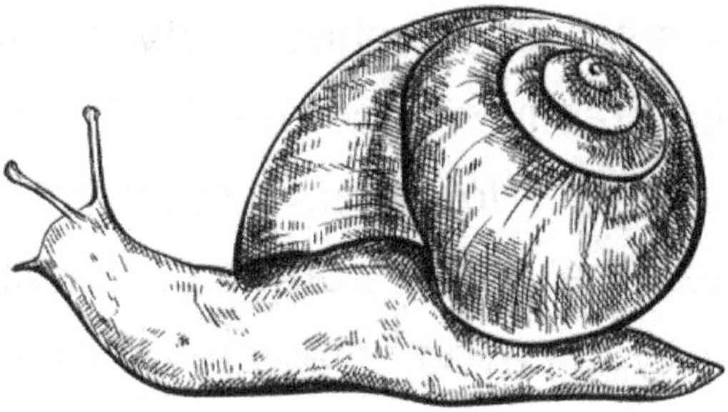

Time in Nature. If nature is left alone, or tended minimally, she usually displays spectacular scenery that lets us know at the deepest level that all is well in the world.

Every tree, every shell, every leaf, every little bird, is perfect. I think this relaxes us in important ways. We can breathe deep for a while, drink in its beauty, and feel that maybe we're a part of it all too.

Sunshine. Get as much sun exposure on your body as possible without burning to increase vitamin D levels. Lack of vitamin D is strongly linked with many health issues. I'm originally from the North West of England, where it was a real treat to see any sun at all. In today's world we've been taught to be afraid of the sun and smear ourselves with toxic sun screen instead. Sunshine is life giving as long as you don't let it burn you. A sun hat and T-shirt make sense in the middle of a hot day, but apart from that, a healthy tan is a wonderful thing.

Hot baths or saunas. The raised temperature acts like a fever to cleanse the body of toxins through the skin.

Organic skin care, toiletries, cleaning and laundry products. Our skin absorbs whatever is in these products so it pays to make them organic and natural.

A clean, clear environment. This helps you think straight and stay calm. Clutter lying around the house distracts us like an endless to-do list constantly calling for our attention and creating stress.

Intermittent fasting (for example, eating one meal a day) is a good way to help your body clear unwanted proteins and toxins, especially after the covid shot.

It's called autophagy and it works like this:

My guess is we've all had times when the fridge is full to bursting. Maybe we had visitors, maybe we were stocking up, but life happens and it all gets out of hand. The vegies wilt, bread grows mould, green slime starts to ooze everywhere and the ham starts to smell.

When you eat three times a day with snacks in between, your poor guts are so overworked trying to process the new food you're eating that similar things can start to happen in your body. Dr Andreas Moritz tells us that 'Undigested food is the greatest source of poisoning in the body.' And goes on to tell us about all the unpleasant things that happen as your food rots in your digestive tract for a couple of days. Digesting food also uses up a lot of your body's energy, which is why you can feel that slump in energy after a big lunch.

I think we've also all had times when the fridge is nearly empty. Maybe we were busy. Maybe it was the end of the month, but there we are at dinner time with half an onion, two old carrots and an unidentified frozen object to work with. We use it all to whip up something surprisingly delicious and give the fridge a spring clean at the same time.

Our ancestors didn't eat all the time, so following their example like this (and staying with nutrient rich foods) not only saves money but allows your body to clean up some of the debris and excess proteins that have accumulated in the system. (I was happy to lose 7 kilos just by eating once a day for a few months. That's a winner in itself for most of us.)

Not eating for four hours before sleep and going to bed on an empty stomach allows the brain to regenerate while we sleep. Eating one meal a day actually boosts the metabolism, gives your body a real chance to give itself a spring clean and reduces the risk of Alzheimer's, ageing, cancer and diabetes. Intermittent fasting is also very different from starving. Starvation just deprives the body of nutrients but with fasting you are eating high nutrient foods less often. These eating plans also break down clots so if you've had the experimental shots then this strategy is crucial. Dr Paul Marik tells us that autophagy breaks down the excess proteins *within* the cells while nattokinase – which we will come to later, breaks down the excess proteins *outside* the cells.

Obviously, this isn't something to inflict on your children or try in pregnancy, although eating good organic food when you're actually hungry will always make sense.

A Health Reset

In general terms, organic raw vegetable juices are a wonderful way to lay the foundations for rebuilding our health. Most of us need more vitamins and minerals in our diet and it's always best to get them from our food if we can.

The living enzymes, vitamins and minerals in organic, raw, freshly juiced vegetables help our digestion and give the system a real break. It takes a lot of energy to digest foods, especially if you're feeling weak in the first place. As the years roll by the hydrochloric acid in the stomach loses strength and, coupled with our tendency to not chew our food thoroughly, can lead to foods not being digested properly. We don't have to try and chew our way through a whole cabbage to get the nutrients from it. We can mix it up with green apple and ginger and drink it all in a glass. Once we invest in a juicer our raw vegetable intake can explode to great healthy baskets full and the fibre can be used in soups and salads, fed to animals or put in the compost. Bottled or pasturised juices will never have the nutrients of fresh juice, which is always best to drink straight away but can be stored in the fridge for a day if necessary.

Type 2 diabetics should avoid all fruits but a raw veggie juice diet like this will allow them to drop their insulin levels to virtually normal over 30 days. Dr Gabriel Cousens writes extensively about this in his book: **'There is a Cure for Diabetes.'**

Interestingly, Chris Wark from **'Chris Beat Cancer'** describes a very similar vegetable juice based diet but with more berries and fruits to help your body recover from cancer in his excellent **'Square One'** program.

For the rest of us, we're always more likely to stick with an eating plan if it tastes good. Fruits are too sweet to drink as juices on their own but freshly made vegie juices or smoothies with beets, carrots, celery, cucumber, spinach, kale, ginger, lemon, dandelion and parsley with granny smith apples, (complete with pips) banana, grapefruit, lemon and berries of all sorts are a good way forward.

There are many juice books and videos but I'll recommend a wonderful one here by Cherie Calbom: **The Juice Lady's Guide to Juicing for Health**. It's clear, concise and simple, with loads of health information and simple recipes.

Cherie lists juices and cleanses for many health issues or parts of the body. You can experiment with the juices but cleanses can be a bit more intense and I suggest tackling these after discussing them with your health practitioner. It's often best to work on one aspect of detox at a time so you are comfortable and the body doesn't feel overwhelmed.

Detox

Let's look at this as if we were cleaning house.

It's fascinating to watch YouTube shows about people cleaning out horribly messy hoarder houses. Most of us clean house regularly and keep away the clutter, mess, mould, ants, cockroaches, mice and other nasties that might want to move in. For whatever reason, these people have lost the battle and let the nasties take over. It's not pretty.

In varying degrees, this is what may be happening in your body. If the toxins build up, your body has to stash them away somewhere so they don't do any harm. This is when your body starts adding fat to store them in. Many of us remember how easy it was to lose weight when we were young and 'clean'. As the years roll by the fat and toxins can build up and suddenly we can't shift that weight as easily any more.

We start clearing at the bottom, as it were, with the trash. Taking out all the trash makes way for the next steps. In your body, you start with the colon.

Colon

Modern diets mean that your colon can get clogged up with clumps of waste that can stay there for years or decades even if you're eating well. You can give yourself an enema, but I'm a great believer in the much more thorough colonic hydrotherapy which gently flushes out far more of those nasties. With a good practitioner there are no downsides. They gently massage the abdominal area to ease out anything that shouldn't be in there. They also check for candida, yeasts and other undesirables. You can actually see old, hardened lumps being flushed away. You don't need a referral. It's only slightly strange, it doesn't hurt, it's clean and quite fascinating. Three sessions over several weeks will allow waste to be flushed away rather than re-absorbed through the toxic layer, and give your body a fresh start and a nice clean colon.

Colon care

Juices: vegetable juices including carrot and celery, minimal fruit

Foods: green leafy vegetables, salads, fermented foods and sauerkraut

Supplements: probiotics

Ask about: psyllium husk powder, bentonite clay

Kidneys

Going back to the house cleaning analogy, Kidneys might be like the kitchen sink and the toilet. We all know that if these are blocked, we can't do much to clean and sort everything else.

Kidneys filter the blood at the rate of 200 litres (over 50 US gallons) every day so waste products and legal and illegal drugs can be removed via the urine. .... pause to get a glass of water ... Kidneys help to control blood pressure and make hormones which produce red blood cells. They balance the acidity and alkalinity of fluids and electrically charged electrolytes in the body.

Kidney care

Start the day with the juice of half a lemon in a glass of hot filtered water.

Juices: Organic parsley, cucumber, asparagus, tomato, coriander leaves, watermelon and ginger.

Foods: organic salads and vegetables

Herbs and supplements: Juniper berry tea, nettle tea, ginger,

Ask about: flushing kidney stones and homeopathy,

Liver

In our house cleaning analogy, the liver would be the one in the middle of it all sorting everything out into piles of keep, store or throw away. The liver is a multi-tasking power house, sorting out your last meal, breaking down toxins, fats and proteins, sifting through what you've eaten and deciding what to send into the blood, what to store in your fat, and what to get rid of. It stores useful minerals and fat-soluble vitamins A, D, E, and gets rid of alcohol and toxins by producing around a litre (2 pints) of bile a day. Apparently around 13% of your blood is in our liver at any one time so it makes sense to look after it.

Liver care

Juices: organic beetroot, cabbage, broccoli, cauliflower, cucumber, carrots, ginger, garlic, lemon, parsley, endive.

Foods: broccoli, sprouts, organic vegetables, mostly raw.

Herbs and supplements: burdock, dandelion, turmeric and milk thistle

Ask about: N-Acetyl-L-Cysteine (NAC), which boosts super anti-oxidant glutathione and helps to detox heavy metals, alcohol and toxins.

Dr Eric Berg explains what NAC is:

https://youtu.be/oPdGOrqTfhA?si=ecH6pVA2roYkOadX

Dr Eric Berg talks about NAC and Glutathione:

https://youtu.be/Ut9_iHFu1uA?si=5LFkoE0OT-79PYkc

Gall :ladder

The gall bladder sits under the liver like a bile storage tank.

Bile is a sticky, yellow-green fluid made by the liver to break down fats into fatty acids so they can be absorbed in the digestive tract.

If we were eating naturally as our ancestors did, with organic vegetables, fish and lean meats, this arrangement would work well for a lifetime. As it is, all those fast foods, sugar, seed oils, pesticides, artificial sweeteners, drugs, preservatives and alcohol that are so much a part of our lives now put a huge strain on everything. They're so toxic that your liver won't even release a lot of them into the body. It'll find a place to stash some of them in our fat cells and it hangs onto the rest of them. They sit there like gravel, silting up perfectly good organs like sand in a polluted river. If you get a gall stone, you'll know about it by the headaches, nausea or sharp pain. Head to the emergency room at once as it can be life threatening. It's wise to *avoid* gall bladder surgery if you possibly can though and head quickly to a natural practitioner for alternatives. You want to hang on to that gall bladder for a lifetime if you can.

Gall Bladder Care

Start the day with the juice of half a lemon in a glass of hot water.

Juices: beetroot. sprouts, carrot, lemon, celery, grapefruit, cabbage, cucumber parsley and apple. (just sweet enough to be palatable is fine unless you are diabetic).

Foods: vegetables and raw salads, vegetable soups.

Herbs and supplements: turmeric, Milk thistle.

Ask about: gall bladder flushes.

Once these main organs are clear, it will be easier to cleanse the rest of the body.

Pancreas

Also tucked under the liver is an important organ called the pancreas. It serves two main functions in the body. It produces digestive enzymes that help break down carbohydrates, proteins and fats in the small intestine. It also produces hormones, including insulin, that are released into the blood to regulate blood sugar levels.

Ideal blood sugar levels are approximately one teaspoon sugar to over 5.5 litres (1.5 gallons) of blood. As processed simple carbohydrates turn into sugar in the digestive system, many of us are eating over **30 teaspoons of sugar a day** or 63 kilos (140 pounds) a year up from just 2.5 kilos (5 pounds) in the early 1900s. The pancreas has a tough job keeping that heap of poisonous sugar out of the blood and making sure everything stays regulated.

Some sugar is burned off as energy, especially if you're working hard all day. A friend recently trained for a 50 kilometre (31 mile) ultra-marathon in the mountains and told me that one of the issues they face is getting enough energy to fuel the body while they're running. If you're not running a marathon today but sitting behind a desk, your mid-morning snack is put straight into storage in the cells. It's the same old story, it's probably sitting in flabby lumps on our belly and hips, but it could be anywhere - around our organs, on our upper arms, or puffing out our cheeks. Once these fat cells are full, they start shutting off any more sugar in a process called **insulin resistance** and it has nowhere to go but our blood.

Back in the blood, it causes even more trouble as diabetes and brings with it a cascade of nasty issues, up to and including amputation.

Intermittent fasting works wonders here as (in the absence of sugars) the body starts burning fat in a process called ketogenesis, which is better all round. Fat burns more slowly and avoids the hunger pangs and energy crashes of burning sugars.

Pancreas care

Drinking eight glasses of filtered water a day can help.

Juices: ginger, cucumber, lettuce, lemon, cabbage, asparagus, wheatgrass

Foods: olive oil, proteins broccoli, kale, raw almonds, black beans

Herbs and supplements: probiotics, turmeric, garlic, magnesium

Ask about: C-60

Lungs

If we return to the house cleaning analogy, the lungs would be the windows. If we were cleaning house, we'd let the fresh air in by throwing open the doors and windows. The lungs remove carbon dioxide waste and deliver oxygen to the blood. If all your spongey little lung cells were laid out flat they would equal the floor space of a small house. If your heart is strong, vigorous exercise helps to keep your lungs working properly. It's a good idea to breathe deeply through the nose and hold the breath for a count of four or five before exhaling. This is calming and creates increased oxygen levels in the blood

Lung Care

Sunshine reduces inflammation and increases melatonin antioxidants.

Juices: Carrot, watercress, lemon, garlic, cucumber, radish.

Foods: organic salads and vegetables, clean sourced fish.

Herbs and Supplements: Vitamin C, Vitamin D, NAC.

Ask About: Infra-red light therapy. Ultra-Violet light

Heart

The heart is the main organ of the cardiovascular system. It pumps blood around the lungs and throughout your body in a network of around 80,000 kilometres (50,000 miles) of blood vessels, delivering oxygen and removing toxins. It works with other body systems to control your heart rate and blood pressure. The food you eat plays a crucial role in keeping your heart healthy, lowering blood pressure and inflammation.

Heart Care

Juices: Organic spinach, kale.

Foods: Avocados, fatty fish like wild salmon, mackerel, sardines and tuna, garlic, organic vegetables and salads, Celtic salt.

Supplements: Quality organic fish oil, Niacin, Co-enzyme Q10. Potassium. Vitamin D.

Ask about: checking your troponin levels to check if you've had a heart attack. The D-deimer test to check for blood clots

:rain

The brain and the spinal cord make up the central nervous system.

The brain weighs about 1.3 kilos or 3lbs and is the ultimate control centre for memory, thought, emotion, touch, movement, breathing, vision, temperature, hunger and everything else in our body. It's the fattiest organ in the body. Good regular chiropractic care is needed to keep the spine, bone structure and nerves in place and working optimally

Brain Care

Juices: tomato, lemon, lettuce, spinach

Foods: wild caught salmon, (unfortunately the vast majority of salmon in Australia is farmed) sardines, cauliflower, kale.

Herbs and supplements: Ginkgo, bacopa and brahmi for blood flow and memory. Spearmint for sharpening the mind, Lemon balm for calming and soothing. B vitamins.

Ask your practitioner about methylene blue.

Thyroid

The thyroid gland is in the neck and produces hormones that affect many functions, menstruation, fertility, mood swings and metabolic rate (the speed with which we process our food). Iodine is a trace mineral essential for the thyroid and often lacking in our diet.

Thyroid care

Juices: radish, lemon, carrot:

Foods: Wild fish, cod, oysters, organ meats, prawns, crab, sardines, cabbage, eggs, seaweeds such as nori, Brazil nuts.

Supplements: nascent iodine.

Ask About: balancing the metabolism.

Skin

The skin is the largest organ of the body, with a total area of about 20 square feet or nearly 2 square metres. It protects us from many things including tiny predators and the elements. It helps regulate body temperature, and permits the sensations of touch, heat, and cold. Skin is mainly protein and fat. It absorbs whatever you put on it so stay away from chemical creams, lotions and perfumes no matter how good they smell. Go natural and organic to keep everything healthy. I love my organic hemp cleanser, and body lotion.

Skin Care

Juices: Capsicum (bell pepper) cucumber, carrot, lemon and pineapple

Foods: Fatty fish, sardines, wild salmon, and mackerel are rich sources of omega-3 fatty acids that help keep skin thick, supple, and moisturized.

Wheat germ. Green and yellow capsicums for vitamin C which helps with collagen production. Pineapple for bromelain. Brazil nuts for selenium to protect against sun damage.

Supplements: Collagen. Vitamin C. Zinc

Ask about: organic tallow skin care

Take Care

In addition, there are three main nasties that we really need to clear from the body that can lodge in various organs: toxic metals, parasites and cancers.

Toxic metals

Toxic metals include lead, cadmium, mercury, arsenic and aluminium. None of these have any place in the body. Aluminium is found in many childhood injections and can lodge in the brain leading to autism and contributing to Alzheimers. No vaccines are properly tested against harmless placebos and should be avoided if we wish to remain healthy.

Consider drinking silica water, juicing carrots, (without the tops) radishes and ginger root.

Expert homeopathy and careful diet are excellent for detoxing aluminium and heavy metals.

Parasites

A parasite is an organism anywhere in the body which may be microscopic but which takes from us but (unlike the good bacteria in our gut) gives nothing back. We are becoming more aware that parasites aren't just something from the third world, or for dogs, cats or livestock. It's interesting that we understand the need to worm these animals regularly but don't think of doing parasite cleanses for ourselves. There is research linking microscopic parasites to a number of diseases including cancer and multiple sclerosis, especially if you have ever lived in a third world country or had pets as a child.

Dr Hulda Clark was a Canadian naturopath who had been speaking about parasites for decades and has several detailed books on the subject.

All this is very relevant at this time as many people used to have healthier bodies which held cancers and parasites in check. Now their immune systems have been weakened by the covid shots and cancers are growing fast. I think the good thing about this is that we have more understanding that this may be an issue and can act fast to turn things around.

Dr Eric Berg lists a number of symptoms, including bloating, itching and fatigue, showing that you might have parasites. He has a number of simple clips and lists some natural supplements needed to combat them.

Dr Lee Merritt, the 'Medical Rebel', speaks in many interviews about possible links between cysts, cancer and parasites. She prefers a more medical based protocol as being more powerful and in all cases a broad net of treatments is needed to catch them all.

Dr Thomas Lodi is an American who now practices in Thailand. He specialises in cancer treatments, has courses on his website and speaks about a cancer/parasite link.

He has an interesting seminar on this and lists a number of detailed anti-parasitic protocols (behind a modest paywall).

Dr. Lodi – Parasites Webinar Replay

Dr Bryan Ardis has a natural parasite cleanse package, 'Freedom, Cleanse and Restore,' on his website which looks easy to navigate:
https://thedrardisshow.com

Global Healing has a quality 'Harmful Organism Cleanse Program'.
https://globalhealing.com

Some of these cleanses need to be timed carefully due to the need to work with the life cycles of these little nasties to make sure they're all dead and won't flare up again. It would be wise to seek expert guidance with these detoxes. Ask your natural therapist about the possibility that this may be an issue.

Cancers

Unfortunately, strange, fast developing turbo-cancers are being seen following covid shots. They usually develop too fast for conventional medical treatments. In the weird world of today this might be seen as a blessing in disguise because you won't be put under pressure to undergo mainstream treatments which may be toxic. Swift and massive action to flood the body with plant juices, anti-oxidants and nutrients is needed if you have a diagnosis after having the shots.

Dr Max Gerson's therapy has been curing people of cancer (and other diseases) consistently since the thirties. The treatment is mostly veggie juices and coffee enemas to alkalize and cleanse the system. (In 1952 Dr Raymond Kaiser, Head of the National Cancer Institute, on seeing Gerson's meticulous records of many cures of advanced cancer cases, said, 'Sometimes these European refugees come over to America and want to make a splash so they go ahead and cure cancer.')

The Gerson Institute still cures patients in San Diego, California.

In 1934, after many years of work, gifted scientist **Royal Raymond Rife** conducted an experiment at the University of Southern California using targeted electromagnetic frequencies to kill cancer. Sixteen terminally ill cancer patients were cured painlessly within four months. A grand dinner was held in his honour. The medical industry then began the systematic destruction of this ground breaking technology, Rife's labs, his records, the equipment he had designed and Rife himself. He died a broken man. Check out the **Spooky 2** Rife frequency machine now used by thousands of people around the world.

Harry Hoxey was curing cancer for decades with recipes derived from Native American recipes and the work continues in Tijuana, Mexico under the name of the Bio Medical Clinic.

Laetrile for B17 (from apricot kernels) was proved in tests by highly regarded Dr Kanematsu Sugiura at the Sloane-Kettering institute to be one of the most effective anti-cancer treatments ever tested on mice. Then it was systematically discredited by that same organisation and later outlawed in the US.

One of the longest-lived communities in the world, the Hunza, has lots of apricots in their diet and prizes the kernels highly. A man's wealth is counted in Apricot trees. Cancer is virtually unknown.

Janette Murray-Wakelin cured herself of breast cancer in her late fifties on a raw wholefoods diet and in 2013 ran 366 consecutive marathons around Australia with her husband on a diet of raw juices and vegetables. I followed their diary on YouTube and have met them both in person. They are now in their seventies. Look for **Running Raw Around Australia** and their documentary: **RAW.**

Dr Stanislaw Burzynski discovered that people with cancer lack certain peptides and pioneered what he called anti-neoplaston cancer treatment in the 80s. **The Burzynski Clinic** in Texas specialises in treating children's brain cancers with no huge toxic side effects and a significant percentage of complete recoveries. Despite this he has been harassed by the Texas Medical Board for three decades. Check the documentary of the same name: **Burzynski**

Check out **'Chris beat Cancer'** for the story of **Chris Wark,** a young man who was diagnosed with advanced colon cancer in 2004 at the age of 26. He chose to cure his bowel cancer naturally and has been studying this form of cancer treatment and sharing his knowledge with other cancer patients ever since. Now in his mid-forties, he looks amazing and his new **'Square One'** program is the clearest and simplest treatment protocol I've ever seen for curing cancer naturally.

Cancer is a disease of toxicity coupled with vitamin and mineral deficiencies, oxygen deficiency (singlet oxygen is especially important) and dehydration so the body can't throw it off any longer.

'Cancer cells and many other imbalances cannot survive in a hydrated, oxygenated, alkaline environment. It's that simple.' **Ed McCabe: Flood Your Body with Oxygen.**

'No disease, including cancer, can exist in an alkaline environment.' **Otto Warburg, 1931 Nobel Prize Winner for cancer discovery.**

Andreas Moritz has some excellent and simple insights about what cancer is doing in the body. It gives clarity on why you are making these changes:

YouTube: https://youtu.be/r18OHoT5Q7o.

Check out the 9-part Documentary **'The Truth about Cancer'** produced by **Ty and Charlene Bollinger.** Steep yourself in this information to really GET that it's real and possible. (Rumble) and website:

https://thetruthaboutcancer.com/category/cancer-treatments/

How to stay healthy? Do some exercise you enjoy every day. Stay off the sugar, processed foods, fried stuff, seed oils, grains, dairy and alcohol. Eat raw organic vegan whenever possible.

Enjoy lots of deep breathing, good air, raw salads, wheatgrass and organic veggie juices with the live plant nutrients still in them.

Drink filtered water, often with lemon juice to alkalize the system. Take an oxygen/mineral supplement, Vitamin D, C, CoQ10, magnesium, omega 3, iodine and B vitamins. And throw in a few of those apricot kernels for good measure ....

If you are already there and have had a diagnosis:

- Buy the **'Square One'** program on line, adapt it to your lifestyle and stick with it.
- Stay calm. Make sure you are exercising every day (if your heart is healthy) Go raw vegan organic with loads of juicing, some fruit, mostly veggies, and clear your environment of as many toxins as possible while you decide what to do.
- Colonic hydrotherapy sessions to clean out the large intestine would be of great benefit

now. (You'll be surprised at what's clogged up in there.)

- Massage and rebounding or even skipping can be good for clearing the lymphatic system and good chiropractic care is always helpful to make sure the body is operating at its peak.
- Meditate.
- Don't let them rush you into chemo treatments and surgery.
- Don't let them frighten you.
- Stay calm.
- Do your research carefully. You have many options.
- Choose the path that's right for you.
- Consider a naturopath or wholistic practitioner who has seen people in your position recover and believes you can too.
- Make a diary of every bit of progress and healing and be grateful and appreciative of every step in the right direction.

Your faith in your own recovery is paramount and you need to find a practitioner who believes in you.

Supplements

It makes sense to flood your body with life-giving organic nutrients at this time. Here is a list of vitamins, minerals and herbs which have been suggested as being specifically helpful on a healing journey after the shots.

If you learn a little about them and what they do, you can discuss them with a natural practitioner and understand which are most suitable for you.

If you are new to the world of natural medicine it might come as a surprise to see plants like 'milk thistle' on the list, but these have been our prime sources of healing for millennia. They are very powerful and more easily absorbed and used by the body than pharmaceutical drugs or even supplements.

The pharmaceutical industry doesn't like natural substances because they can't be patented and it's the expensive newly patented drugs that make for the biggest profits.

We often find that natural plants or remedies that should be freely available from our own gardens are outlawed or less common than they should be.

Ethical growers often have to dodge many unhelpful regulations and this makes many natural remedies more expensive than they should be.

I suspect that those colourful traditional country cottage gardens we can see on Pinterest were actually full of medicinal herbs, seeds and flowers which were carefully harvested and preserved for use over the year.

Supplements are one of the simplest ways you can start to support your body if you didn't get an injection and your symptoms are very mild.

Immune boosting vitamins

Vitamin C - is an immune booster and an antioxidant. It can protect your body from the toxins that cause inflammation.

Found naturally in citrus fruits and broccoli, cauliflower and brussels sprouts.

Vitamin D3 - is a fat-soluble vitamin that can help protect against flu like illness by boosting levels of natural antibiotics. Vitamin D3 has receptors in almost every cell in the human body.

Found naturally in sunshine.

Vitamin K2 - is also fat soluble and a great companion to take with vitamin D3 to help strengthen the immune system.

Found naturally in green leafy vegetables

Zinc - is important for cell growth and division, immune function, wound healing and fighting off infection.

Found naturally in oysters, liver, beans and lentils.

Quercetin - is a powerful anti-inflammatory. It opens the cells and becomes even more powerful when teamed with zinc. It helps to drive the zinc deep into the cell where it's most needed.

Found naturally in citrus fruits, parsley, onions.

Magnesium – is a mineral that is essential for healthy muscles, nerves, bones and blood sugar levels and is involved in hundreds of biochemical reactions in your body, including:

Energy creation: converting food into energy.

Protein formation: creating new proteins from amino acids.

Gene maintenance: helping create and repair DNA and RNA.

Muscle movements: aiding in muscle contraction and relaxation.

Nervous system regulation: regulating the neurotransmitters which send messages throughout your brain and nervous system.

Found naturally in leafy greens, whole grains, nuts.

Complex B vitamins - including B12 and B6 are important for a healthy immune response. B6 is vital in supporting biochemical reactions in the immune system to produce white blood cells and T- cells. These are the cells that are responsible for fighting off invaders like viruses and bacteria. It is important that people who don't eat meat or fish supplement with B vitamins and B12 in particular.

Found naturally in liver, beef

Vitamin E - is a powerful anti-oxidant which plays a part in over 200 biochemical reactions in the body. It supports the immune system to help fight off infection.

Found naturally in sunflower seeds, almonds, hazelnuts.

Vitamin A is important for the immune system and eye health. It is a potent anti-oxidant which fights infection and can help to reduce the risk of some forms of cancer.

Found naturally in cod liver oil, liver, sweet potato.

Nattokinase - is fermented from soy beans and has been eaten for many years in Japan. It's an enzyme which has anti-clotting effects and dismantles proteins into smaller fragments such as amino acids.

The covid shots appear to program your own body to produce the toxic spike proteins that seem to do most of the damage.

Nattokinase is highly effective in breaking down these unwanted proteins, cleaning and clearing the blood of people who have been injected or are suffering with 'long covid'.

Bromelain - is made from pineapples. It's an enzyme (catalyst) that eases inflammation and swelling. Research has also shown that it too helps to break down the spike proteins, blood clots, oedema (water retention) and swelling. We all know that if we eat a lot of fresh pineapple, our mouths can become strangely sensitive, almost as if a layer of cells were being removed, and I believe this is a sign of this protein breakdown effect.

Curcumin - is the active ingredient in turmeric. It's well known for its powerful anti-inflammatory properties. People damaged by the shots have high amounts of inflammation so curcumin is the ideal partner in this three- pronged base protocol approach to treating vaccine injury.

Ivermectin - is an anti-parasitic drug which has been used safely since its discovery and development in the late seventies. Its pharmaceutical patent had expired, so it was being produced around the world for a few cents a packet. It was found to be effective in covid relief protocols but may also have contraceptive properties.

NAC N-acetylcysteine - helps with the production of super anti-oxidant **glutathione** and is a major detoxifier of many unwanted substances, such as alcohol and prescription drugs.

Found naturally in Lentils, beans, spinach, salmon, tuna

Aloe Vera - is a powerful addition to juices and smoothies to promote healing of the skin and gut.

Milk Thistle - is an anti-oxidant and which helps with liver function and gall bladder disorders.

Activated Charcoal - This cleanses the blood of toxins just as it cleanses the water in your filter. It should be taken consistently.

Organic real pine needle tea - is high in vitamin C and other substances which may help to neutralize spike protein.

Dandelion root tea - can be made from the dandelions in your garden unless you spray them with chemicals. As any gardener knows, dandelions have very long roots which draw potent nutrients from deep underground.

Iodine - (I take nascent iodine from Miracle Products and like the way it disperses immediately into water. I think of it doing the same thing in my body, heading quickly to wherever it's needed)

C60 molecule - from charcoal doubled the life-span of rats in lab tests. It's good as an anti-ageing supplement as it boosts autophagy and the cleaning up of old cells,

Hydroxychloroquine - has been used safely since the 1960s to treat malaria and auto-immune diseases such as lupus and inflammatory arthritis. It has been found to be very effective in covid relief protocols.

Chlorophyll - binds to carcinogens such as aflatoxin which is found in peanuts and stored grains.

Coriander - Coriander leaves are a great cleanser

Wheatgrass - a superfood packed with nutrients and anti-oxidants

Vital Greens - an Australian brand which includes a huge variety of dried ground healthy greens in a handy pack.

St John's Wort - relieves depression and anxiety.

Ginger - stimulates the digestive tract.

Burdock root - removes toxins from the blood

Brahmi Bacopa (monniera) - enhances brain function and reduces stress levels. Some years ago, I was chatting to a fellow camper at a caravan site and she shared with me how her memory was fading to the point that she was reluctant to go out. She started taking this ayurvedic herb and it all came back, quickly and clearly. She was as sharp as a tack, and spoke with the enthusiasm of someone sharing an important and helpful insight.

I never forgot the herb or the story.

Gingko Biloba - helps brain function and reduces inflammation.

Olive leaf extract - reduces cardiovascular risk and inflammation.

Essiac Tea - a famous blend of herbs said to kill cancer and remove toxins.

Methylene Blue - boosts the mitochondria, improves energy levels, helps with urinary tract infections and brain function.

EDTA is used in chelation therapies which draw toxins such as lead, arsenic, aluminium, or mercury, from the body. It used to be a comparatively rare treatment which was done intravenously but it is now available as drops and even creams. It should always be done with expert guidance as it can also remove valuable nutrients.

Dr Eric Berg outlines how EDTA works to remove certain toxins from the body and emphasises the need for expert guidance in this process. *https://youtu.be/sFH-0Uu24-c?si=DSCCAqtjjcfSHMz-*

Fenbendazole - an anti-parasitic medication.

Niclosamide - an anti-parasitic medication.

Chlorine Dioxide

Chlorine dioxide - is worth a special mention. It has been used around the world for nearly 100 years as a highly effective water purifier. It isn't bleach. It is an oxidising biocide that is almost 100% effective against viruses, bacteria, fungi, moulds, mites, parasites, biofilms and other harmful organisms. It evaporates without residue or trace and is widely used in food and water treatment industries for this reason. Most of these nasties are anaerobic and simply can't survive in an oxygen rich environment.

In 1996 a gold prospector was leading a mining expedition in the jungles of South America. They were carrying chlorine dioxide as a water purifier. Two of his men had come down with malaria. In the middle of nowhere with two very sick or dying men and nothing to lose, he mixed a couple of drops of the chlorine dioxide solution in water and gave it to them. Within a few hours they were well, strong, and ready to set off again. It was as if he had given them a **miracle mineral solution**.

Since then, similar results have been seen with a huge array of diseases and conditions, including malaria, In turn, this wonderful discovery has thrown the pharmaceutical industry into a panic. Instead of researching these thousands of testimonials so we could all benefit at minimal cost, the pharmaceutical industry has preferred to demonise cheap and simple treatments.

If people were to find out that, with **correct and careful dosing,** they could heal themselves quickly for a few dollars, the pharmaceutical industry might become virtually obsolete. Is this why there are so many dire warnings about taking chlorine dioxide and MMS (miracle mineral solution) around the internet, even while they endorse it for cleaning apples, sterilizing food production machinery or operating theatre instruments?

The Universal Antidote documentary: The Universal Antidote – The Science and Story of Chlorine Dioxide

A lot of these products aren't cheap, especially if they come from the US. With supplements and nutrients you often get what you pay for. Discernment is key. Generally the brands offered by professional naturopaths are more potent, more likely to be balanced and better for you. than cheap supermarket brands. This is an important investment in your health and you owe it to yourself not to skimp on it.

Our miraculous bodies are incredibly complex and people suffering symptoms after the shots really do need a trusted wholistic practitioner to lead them back to health.

Websites

This is a list of the main websites dealing with post covid jab issues.

Many of the doctors mentioned in these websites were at the top of their field of expertise in the pre-covid era and many have resigned or been sacked for speaking out against damaging covid shots. This is now such a common story it's a badge of honour and gives us an indication of their integrity and willingness to genuinely help people.

I suggest that you familiarise yourself with these websites and use your new knowledge to find your own individual practitioner.

The Zelenko Protocols

Dr Vladimir Zelenko was a family doctor in New York and one of the first doctors to respond to the covid era in 2020 by putting together a number of successful protocols to prevent and ease symptoms of the original covid infections. Early treatment has always been a cornerstone of good medicine so people are treated *long before* symptoms become distressing, urgent and life threatening.

At the time, people around the world were being told that there was no early treatment and that they should go home and do nothing until they couldn't breathe. Many people died because of this delay.

Dr Zelenko was one of many doctors around the world who were valiantly trying to share information about simple, effective early treatments. Sadly **Dr Zelenko** died of cancer in 2022 but the website is still a wealth of information on covid prevention and treatments.

https://vladimirzelenkomd.com/treatment-protocol/

World Council
For Health

World Council for Health:

Founded in 2021, this is an independent global coalition of health advocates, doctors, innovators and activists who are sharing a wealth of knowledge in 16 languages to help people regain their health.

The website is very clear and simple, has some great video presentations and many suggestions for supplements and protocols that may help you to reverse the damage with the help of your chosen practitioner. I believe this website is showing us a glimpse of what health care may look like in the future. You may find the page below (which is constantly being updated as new information comes to light) to be especially useful:

https://worldcouncilforhealth.org

https://worldcouncilforhealth.org/resources/spike-protein-detox-guide/

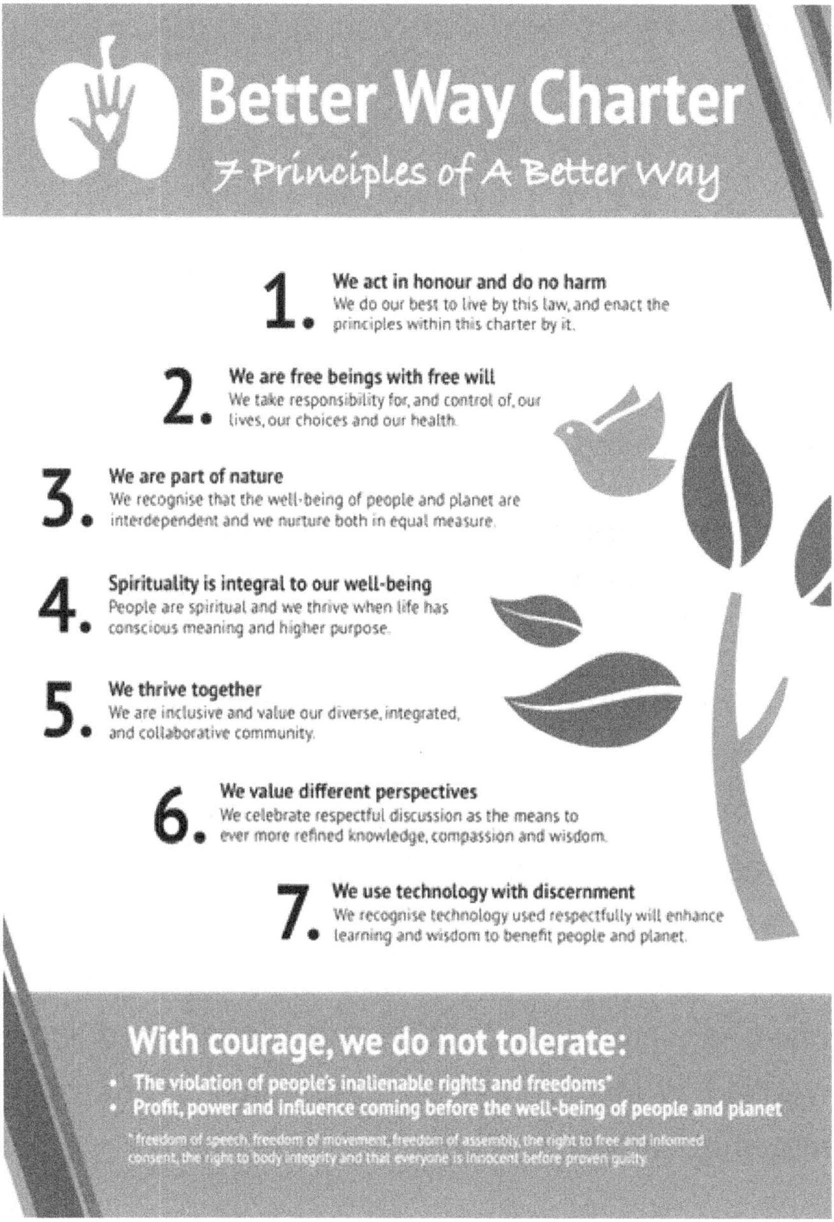
Better Way Charter
7 Principles of A Better Way
1. We act in honour and do no harm
We do our best to live by this law, and enact the principles within this charter by it.
2. We are free beings with free will
We take responsibility for, and control of, our lives, our choices and our health.
3. We are part of nature
We recognise that the well-being of people and planet are interdependent and we nurture both in equal measure.
4. Spirituality is integral to our well-being
People are spiritual and we thrive when life has conscious meaning and higher purpose.
5. We thrive together
We are inclusive and value our diverse, integrated, and collaborative community.
6. We value different perspectives
We celebrate respectful discussion as the means to ever more refined knowledge, compassion and wisdom.
7. We use technology with discernment
We recognise technology used respectfully will enhance learning and wisdom to benefit people and planet.
With courage, we do not tolerate:
• The violation of people's inalienable rights and freedoms*
• Profit, power and influence coming before the well-being of people and planet
* freedom of speech, freedom of movement, freedom of assembly, the right to free and informed consent, the right to body integrity and that everyone is innocent before proven guilty

WORLD OF WELLNESS
INTERNATIONAL

WOW: World of Wellness

Dr Ian Brighthope is the holistic doctor who founded the **Australasian College of Nutritional and Environmental** Medicine in Australia in the '80s. He stepped up again to create **World of Wellness International** in response to the lockdowns of the covid era. It's a not-for-profit organisation to represent the health, wellbeing, human rights and peaceful interests of people everywhere.

It is allied with the **World Council for Health** and offers advice, education and support for doctors wanting to incorporate a holistic style of medicine into their practice. There is a referral service for people seeking medical advice from a doctor who is open to natural treatments.

The group offers consultations with political and industry leaders about the effectiveness of natural therapies so they can be used in new health policies. Unfortunately, cheap and simple preventive measures are often not well received by pharmaceutical industries or politicians.

Dr Brighthope speaks about nutrition and diet as the basic building blocks of health that can help protect us against severe and acute diseases.

https://wowintl.org/#

The FLCCC Alliance

The Front Line Covid 19 Critical Care Alliance was founded in March 2020 by a group of leading critical care specialists including **Dr Paul Marik** and **Dr Pierre Kory.**

The Front Line COVID-19 Critical Care Alliance (FLCCC) is dedicated to the prevention and treatment of covid, especially after the shots. It also aims to help patients take charge of other areas of their health. I encourage you to read the protocols carefully, but remember that even if your symptoms after taking the shots are mild, you will need the guidance and partnership of a naturopath or trusted natural health practitioner. This organization is predominantly US based.

https://covid19criticalcare.com/

The Wellness Company

The Wellness Company is in this line up in recognition of the courageous work of world-renowned cardiologist **Dr Peter McCullough** and obstetrician **Dr James Thorp,** both of whom have spoken out fearlessly in the covid era. They are both now on **The Wellness Company's** medical board.

Dr Peter McCullough is one of the most published doctors in the world, specialising in heart health and the transmission of disease.

He has put forward a basic natural formula he believes is most effective for clearing the body of excess proteins, which seem to be one of the main issues. Similar protocols can be found on the other websites listed and the case histories featured later in this book have shown us that these protocols are working.

https://www.twc.health/

Dr Peter McCullough is an outspoken cardiologist and epidemiologist. Based on his research so far, this is his suggested natural spike detox base protocol. He suggests staying on it for 12 months.

Nattokinase: 100 milligrams
- twice a day without food.
Bromelain: 500 milligrams - once a day without food.
Curcumin: 500 milligrams - twice a day.

A nutrient rich diet and intermittent fasting are also beneficial

THE dr.ardis SHOW

Dr Bryan Ardis has some interesting research which seems to be an important piece of the puzzle and which deserves a spot in this line up.

While we were being told stories about bats and pangolins getting together in Chinese live animal markets it seems that research with various lethal snake venoms has been carried out by US health authorities for decades. It's possible to duplicate a range of snake venoms artificially to manufacture them on a large scale and their various effects sound suspiciously like the symptoms of covid, long covid, covid shots and remdesivir. These include respiratory distress, clotting, loss of taste and smell, paralysis and organ failure.

He also tells us that nicotine, (which is found in several vegetables as well as tobacco leaves,) is actually a nutrient when used on its own and helps to block the receptors in the brain which take up these toxins. Apparently, smokers didn't usually suffer from covid. No-one is recommending taking up smoking, but for some people, especially those with neurological issues, a nicotine patch or nicotine gum might be worth trying. Start with a small piece and work up. (This is not medical advice)

Bryan tells us that from his investigation into government funded research it appears that this severe type of poisoning seems to be lessened by **N Acetyl Cysteine, Vitamin C, Glutathione and EDTA.** All of these are mentioned in the book

He has many conversations with eminent doctors on this subject and this particular line-up of treatments would certainly be worth investigating if other treatments don't work as normal.

Bryan Ardis speaks about some of his research and gives some simple common sense health precautions to David and Stacey Whited on **Flyover** *https://rumble.com/v3kst6j-dr.-bryan-ardis-the-10-things-you-need-to-know.html*

He has a range of supplements available on his website:

https://thedrardisshow.com

Dr. Lee Merritt
The Medical Rebel

The Medical Rebel

Lee Merritt is a retired surgeon, deep thinker and self-styled medical rebel who is well worth checking out. She believes that microscopic parasites may be the source of many of our issues, including cancers, especially after covid injections and has a number of in-depth interviews and protocols on this topic. It's interesting to note here that both Ivermectin and Hydroxychloroquine are both anti-parasitic medications.

https://www.drleemerritt.com/

SQUARE ONE
healing cancer
coaching program

Chris Wark was diagnosed with advanced colon cancer at the age of 26 in 2004. After an initial surgery he chose to cure his bowel cancer naturally and has been studying effective cancer protocols and sharing his knowledge with other cancer patients ever since. Now in his mid-forties, he looks amazing, he's very relatable and he brings his vast wealth of insight and knowledge into his new on line 'Square One' program.

The price is reasonable and it's the clearest and simplest treatment protocol I've ever seen for curing cancer naturally in a way that works for you.

https://www.chrisbeatcancer.com

https://sq1.chrisbeatcancer.com

Spooky2

Spooky 2 frequency machine.

Healing with coherent frequencies is becoming more accepted all the time. This machine is named after a quote of **Albert Einstein** who spoke about 'Spooky action at a distance'. It's based on the brilliant healing work of **Royal Raymond Rife**. Rife's frequency machine healed many advanced cancer patients, was celebrated at the highest levels, then quickly destroyed by the medical establishment of the day.

Everything has a frequency: from healthy tissue to the common cold, staph infections or parasites. Rife and the companies who have developed his machine in recent times have programmed **hundreds** of unwanted conditions into the device, which can clear them from your body as you sleep. Discoveries that cure people quickly and painlessly have never been popular with the health industry. **John White,**

the designer of this machine speaks in his quiet, understated manner about coherent frequency healing. He explains that frequencies are normally scattered, and compares this to being surrounded by a crowd of shouting children and being unable to even hear what they're saying, let alone respond to them. If you can calm them down and get them to say one thing at a time, then you can understand and reply sensibly to them so everyone is happier. There are other frequency machines on the market, but I would check this one out first.
https://wwwspooky2.com

Studying these websites carefully will give you many insights on how to choose the best local practitioner for your needs. The websites are updated as new information comes to light and there is a vast wealth of information here that can help you to heal.

How to choose a practitioner:

The person who injected you with this wildly experimental shot, or refused to believe you had been damaged by it, is unlikely to be able to help you now. You will need to find a naturopath or wholistic doctor who is aware of the effects the shots are having on the population around the world. Remember that many practitioners are able to work on Zoom from anywhere in the world which will give you a lot more choice.

Personal contact might be preferable, but isn't always necessary.

Study these pages and the websites carefully. Read the articles and follow up on some of the doctors you have seen on there. Check out what they are saying and which other professionals and pages they hang out with. This is how you empower yourself.

Check out the links at the back of the book.

If you prefer to work with a local practitioner, ask for recommendations on the **World of Wellness** website (which is Australian based), your local health food store, organic market, or aware friends.

Put together a list of the medications and vaccines you have taken recently, together with manufacturer names, dates and batch numbers if you can. Start a diary with notes of treatments and symptoms.

Write out at least three questions based on what you have learned. Make sure you know and understand the correct answer to at least one of the questions.

Now you have your questions about your healing, check out your local natural practitioners. You may be working closely with them for many months so it's important that you trust and feel comfortable with them.

It's really like a job interview, with you as the employer. Choose a good practitioner just as you might choose a good vehicle mechanic or hairdresser.

Visit the practitioners, tell them of your intention to heal and ask your questions. You might mention the work of **Dr Peter McCullough, Dr Pierre Kory, Dr Paul Marik, Dr Ryan Cole or Dr Ian Brighthope.** Have they heard of these people? Do they know their work? If they don't recognise a couple of these names at once, I suggest that you're in the wrong place.

Show them this book. If they show no interest and become defensive about the fact that you are educating yourself, I suggest that you're in the wrong place.

You are looking for practitioners who are willing to have an open and honest conversation with you and who recognise and welcome the insights of groups such as the **World Council for Health, World of Wellness, or the Front Line Covid Critical Care Alliance. (FLCCC).**

These are some of the doctors at the leading edge of covid and covid injection recovery. **If there are going to be any breakthrough treatments in this field, these people are likely to know about it first.**

Once you've established that the practitioner is knowledgeable, do they listen to you? Do they seem confident? Do they have some answers? Do they even know the questions? Do they take the time to explain things to you? What tests are they suggesting and why? You're a lot better educated now than you used to be. Do you think they know what they are talking about? Can you trust them? Do you feel comfortable with them?

Once you find your practitioner, and agree on a course of treatment, it makes sense to invest in the items they recommend and follow all their instructions as closely as you can. Record your sessions with them so you can remember what they say. Continue your diary notes to track products, dosing, emotional wellbeing and physical improvements. Give yourself a mark out of ten for how you feel each day. It might be that your symptoms and direction change along the journey to recovery and it's certainly possible that new techniques and healing modalities will be found along the way.

Tests you might ask about:

- D-Dimer test for blood clots
- Tryponin test for heart damage
- Blood testing for nutrient levels
- **Live blood analysis** to see the quality of your cells. A pinprick of your blood is taken and immediately put on a microscope slide so you can check on your live blood cells moving around on the computer screen.

I like this idea but my naturopath friends assure me that it's not always easy to obtain or interpret an accurate picture with basic skills and equipment. If you are keen to do this sort of test, I encourage you to find a career specialist in the field with high quality, specialised equipment and good testimonials.

Pregnancy

Extra special care will always be needed if you are pregnant or hoping to fall pregnant. If you or your partner have had any vaccines, especially **Gardasil** (the notorious human papiloma virus vaccine) or the covid shots, it is a very good idea for **both of you** to cleanse, detoxify, and check nutrient levels and sexual health **before** planning a pregnancy.

Gardasil 9 toxicity may be removed from the body with a specialised homeopathic detox.

Unfortunately, both covid and Gardasil shots are known to affect your ability to fall pregnant, sustain a pregnancy to full term and give birth to a healthy baby. Both these shots can have an impact on sperm quality and it's as well to be aware of this information with a thorough reproductive health check **before** you learn slowly the hard way through harsh personal experience. It is now well documented and increasingly well known that the healthiest babies of all time are born naturally, have had no injections of any kind, including in the womb, and are breast fed for over 6 months.

Once again, nature knows best.

No vaccines of any kind are tested for safety in pregnancy. Over 35 years ago when I had my children, advice from **every** doctor and **every** baby book was very clear: Don't drink alcohol, take a pill, smoke or have a vaccine if you want the best for your baby.

Wise advice then. Wise advice now.

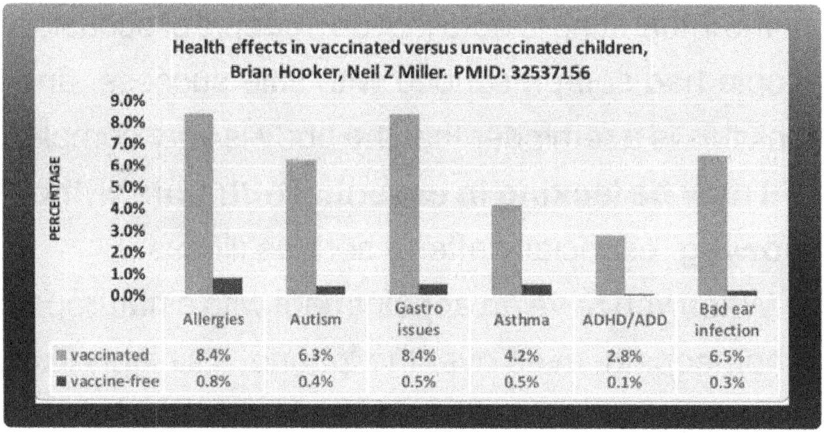

Case Studies

What's working?

These results speak for themselves. I am so grateful to these professionals for sharing their successful treatments in these case histories. I think it gives us all hope that you can recover from these strange afflictions and regain your health naturally.

It is interesting to note that on a couple of occasions people had self-prescribed with little success, and I think this is a reminder that the body is very complex. **You may be lacking in essential nutrients without knowing,** especially after a serious illness.

When you have an appointment with a naturopath or homeopath, even over the 'phone, it's highly likely that your first consultation will be for an hour, in which she or he will ask many questions about the signs and symptoms of your health history. While you are talking, they will be listening carefully for clues and making notes so they can help you better. The following appointments are likely to be for 30-45 minutes as every improvement and change in your condition is carefully noted.

As they work with you to strengthen the body, any changes will not be a quick fix, but a gradual improvement which may take weeks.

It is also clear from one of these case histories in particular that these professionals will strongly recommend you visit a doctor or an accident and emergency department if they consider that urgent medical intervention is needed.

If you are suffering anything remotely as severely as these patients, we advise you to seek independent professional, naturopathic or homeopathic advice and guidance to steer you safely through

Lee Clarke, Naturopath

Advanced Diploma in Applied Health Science, Diploma in Iridology, Diploma in Mechanotherapy (massage, lymph drainage, tension release and movement) Certificate in Homeopathy

N.D Dip.Irid Dip.Mech Cert.Hom

https://www.thebodyofnaturalhealth.com.au

Case Study 1: Injured from 2 doses of the Pfizer Injection

A 32 year-old man came to me for help after a vaccine injury. He told me he did not want to take the vaccine but was mandated to do so to keep his job.

He said that before taking the shot he was in the best condition of his life. He was very fit, health conscious and had no underlying medical conditions. He ate well, didn't smoke or drink and had plenty of energy for a busy job, active sports and regular workouts at the gym.

After the 2nd Pfizer injection things took a severe turn and he ended up in hospital for a week.

Symptoms included chest pain, arrhythmia, (irregular heartbeat) shortness of breath, debilitating chronic fatigue and severe digestive issues. He was diagnosed with pericarditis and myocarditis.

The doctors at the hospital treated some of these symptoms which then settled down somewhat, sent him home and told him he just needed rest.

Once home he continued to have ongoing symptoms. He sought help from different doctors to no avail. Some things did improve slightly but he had ongoing issues that prevented him from doing all the things he had enjoyed before.

After 18 months of this he was referred to me. I told him about **Dr Peter McCullough**, who is a world-renowned cardiologist and a group of other doctors from around the world who had been having great success with healing the vaccine injured with their all-natural protocol. I sent him a link to a video for him to watch:

Dr Peter McCullough: *How to Detox Spike Protein from Body (August 2023) (onedaymd.com)*

And also links of where he could buy the products here in Australia.

Doctor's Best Nattokinase 2000 FU 90c - My Health Food Shop

Source Naturals Bromelain 500mg 60c - My Health Food Shop

Herbs of Gold Bio Curcumin 5400 60t - My Health Food Shop

The base protocol consists of three products:-

Nattokinase	2000IU twice per day (100mg)
Bromelain	500mg once per day
Curcumin	500mg twice per day

We looked at these supplements earlier in the book, but they seem to have a pivotal role in many treatments so here they are again:

***Nattokinase** is fermented from soy beans and has been used for many years in Japan. It's an enzyme which splits proteins down into smaller fragments such as amino acids and has anti-clotting effects. It has shown great results in breaking down the spike proteins that do most of the damage from both the covid shots and the covid illness itself. The covid shots appear* *to program your own body to produce toxic spike proteins. Nattokinase is highly effective in breaking down these unwanted proteins, cleansing and clearing the blood of people who have been injected.*

***Bromelain** is made from pineapples. It's an enzyme (catalyst) that eases inflammation and swelling. Research has also shown that it too helps to break down the spike proteins, blood clots, oedema (water retention) and swelling. We all know that if we eat a lot of fresh pineapple, our mouth can become sensitive and I wonder if this is a sign of this protein breakdown effect.*

***Curcumin** is the active ingredient in turmeric. It's well known for its powerful anti-inflammatory properties. Those people damaged by the shots have high amounts of inflammation so curcumin is the ideal partner in this three-pronged approach to treating vaccine injury.*

While he was waiting for these products to arrive, I started him on some targeted high-strength, high-dose vitamin, mineral and herbal blends to address each of his symptoms and improve systems that were affected, and he started to see some good improvements.

It was really after the other products arrived and he started taking them that he saw a remarkable improvement in a very short time. Within 4 weeks of commencing the treatments all of his issues were resolved.

This allowed me to reduce each of the vitamin and mineral products as each system improved. suggested to him to continues on the **base spike protocol** for at least 3 months as has been recommended, which he was more than happy to do.

Case Study 2: Vaccine injured after one Pfizer injection

A 45 year-old woman was referred to me after becoming ill following just one Pfizer shot.

Her symptoms included chronic fatigue and severe brain fog. She was experiencing what she described as electric shock sensations that would happen randomly in different parts of her body.

She had constant nausea and had severe bouts of vomiting over many months and was unable to keep food down. The doctors didn't know what was wrong with her and had prescribed different drugs including many rounds of antibiotics. These either made little difference or in some instances, made her feel worse.

I advised her to order the 3-part protocol of nattokinase, bromelain and curcumin. While she was waiting for that to arrive, I started her on a gut health protocol to help repair her digestive tract and re-populate the microbiome that was clearly destroyed by both the shot and the antibiotics. Our aim was to help her keep food down to improve the chronic fatigue symptoms and build up her strength and energy.

I put her on some combination supplements to help calm down the inflammation of the nervous system which was causing the electric shock type symptoms.

After two weeks she was starting to feel somewhat better. The nausea easing up and she was starting to keep food down. Her fatigue was not quite so bad but the brain fog remained.

She then added Peter McCullough's Nattokinase, Bromelain and Curcumin protocol to the treatment and started to see huge improvements over the next few weeks. She is now over 90 percent recovered and continuing to improve each day. She will continue with the treatment until her recovery is complete.

It has been wonderful for me to have access to these protocols and see results like this. It should give us all hope that we can really help people regain their health. I'm so grateful to Dr McCullough who has searched constantly for real treatments and shared the information freely in the most trying of times.

Patricia Vandenberg-Smith

Bachelor of Health Science, Naturopathy. Diploma of Homeopathy
(BHSci Nat). Dip.Hom
https://www.journeytohealth.com.au

Case Study 1: Healing after two Pfizer shots

My patient was a 28 year-old male detective. He was very fit and active before taking the jab. He was not worried about taking it at the time, but it was required to keep his job.

7th October 2021 - First Pfizer Injection

First Pfizer injection at his doctor's office. His arm was sore and he felt light headed, but he thought nothing about it. That evening he felt a little tightness in his chest and was very fatigued, he went to bed very early and was fine the next morning. For the next week the days were normal. He was just a little more tired than usual, but he was extremely tired in the evening with a feeling of constriction in his chest.

9th October 2021 - Second Pfizer injection.
He asked his doctor if his symptoms had anything to do with the vaccine. He was told *'of course not'* so he went ahead with his second shot. He had the same symptoms as before: constriction and fatigue at night. Seven days later, after a high stress day at work, he went to the hospital with severe tightness in his chest and difficulty breathing.

He had an ECG/ (an electro-cardiogram to check heart function) blood testing and an x-ray, He was told that everything was fine and that he had an anxiety/panic attack. He told them he knew what anxiety and panic felt like and this was nothing like it. He was told to take Nurofen (an over-the-counter anti-inflammatory and pain killer) and go home. The discomfort and pain continued overnight and he went back to the hospital again. He was *again* told to go home and take Nurofen. He later went back to hospital for the third time because he felt freezing cold in the chest, had chest pain and his heart rate was up to 72 bpm (beats per minute.) from his normal rate of 55-60 bpm. He was diagnosed with pericarditis and prescribed Colchicine and Oxycodone for treatment and long-term pain relief.

He continued to visit his doctor and the hospital but the tightness in his chest continued; the fatigue was overwhelming, and his heart rate was terrifying with any kind of exertion. He knew this was a reaction to the vaccination despite constantly being told it had nothing to do with it.

He had never been to a Naturopath before, but I was recommended as a Naturopath who specialised in vaccine reactions, and he was desperate to try anything to regain his health.

26th October 2021 - 1st phone consultation.

He was too weak to leave his home. After discussing his symptoms, I prescribed both homeopathic and naturopathic remedies.

In homeopathy we prescribe a remedy to produce the same symptoms as the 'dis-ease'. We study the individual history very carefully beforehand and prescribe accordingly. Homeopathics are so diluted that you only get the vibration of the substance that caused the problem. It sounds counter intuitive, but ***like cures like.***

The symptoms caused by a substance can be healed or removed by the homeopathic version.

Homeopathy has proved itself over two centuries and in recent decades is well known to be very helpful in healing damage caused by normal vaccinations.

My Treatment

- Pfizer 200c: homeopathic potency – every second night
- Aconite 200c: homeopathic - twice a day. (Anti-inflammatory)
- Nattokinase: three times a day
- N-Acetyl Cysteine: 1 teaspoon - twice a day. (this boosts the potent antioxidant, glutathione)
- Mushroom herbal complex, 1 teaspoon - three times a day
- Quercetin: twice a day (an anti-inflammatory which opens the cells to allow the supplements to do their work.)

9th November 2021 - 2nd consultation.

He was still extremely fatigued, but his chest pain had eased. His heart rate was closer to normal. He had some headaches and was still unable to work.

My Treatment

- Pfizer 1M potency homeopathic - every second night
- Aconite 200c homeopathic - twice a day (anti-inflammatory)
- Nattokinase: twice a day (to break down unwanted proteins)
- High dose hawthorn supplement (to protect the heart and slow and steady the heartbeat.)
- CoQ10 – 3 per day (an anti-oxidant to help boost energy levels)
- Quercetin: once a day (an anti-inflammatory which opens the cells to allow the supplements to do their work.)
- Herbal formula for fatigue – every morning

7th December 2021 - 3rd consultation.

He had seen the heart specialist again, and was given the 'all clear' but also given a prescription for high cholesterol, blood pressure medication and blood thinners for 'prevention of another incidence'. The specialist scoffed at him when he said that he believed he had a vaccine reaction and that a naturopath was helping him to return to health.

Although things had improved a lot, he was still very tired sometimes. He asked the specialist if he could have a sick note to present to work. He was told it wasn't necessary and that he was fine to go back to work once he started the new medications.

My Treatment

- Pfizer 10M homeopathic: twice a week
- Plus continued prior prescription

18 December 2021 - 4th consultation.

He was feeling much better. We agreed he should continue on the supplements I had prescribed through the Christmas break and into the new year.

I received a text from him in the new year of 2022 telling me how very grateful he was for my heartfelt support, for believing him when he told me he was vaccine injured, and for giving him his health back.

Case Study 2: Healing after Pfizer and Novavax

My patient was a 35yr old female receptionist. She was a regular at the gym 3 times a week. She was required to have the vaccine for work and took the

Pfizer vaccine twice, 8 weeks apart. She told me that she was quite sick after each shot with headaches, nausea and fatigue. She spoke to her doctor about getting an exemption from any further vaccinations, if they were demanded, and was told she had no grounds for an exemption. She was required to take a booster shot to continue working at her office so she tried the Novavax shot this time.

She was sick for weeks. She had chest x-rays, and a D-dimer test (which checks for blood clotting). These were found to be clear, full blood tests showed a low white cell count (*Neutrophils* are the most common type of white blood cells and they help to protect the body from infection. *Neutropenia,* or low white cell count, can be caused by repeated infections, autoimmune disease, or cancer treatments and it increases the risk of severe infections.)

12th May 2022 - 1st online consultation.

Her symptoms were extreme chest heaviness, debilitating fatigue and a constant throbbing headache. She felt that the doctor wasn't listening to her concerns, especially when he told her that the symptoms she was experiencing were due to anxiety.

My Treatment

- Pfizer 200c homeopathic twice a week for 2 weeks,
- Pfizer 1M homeopathic twice a week for 2 weeks
- High dose serrapeptase twice a day. (This breaks down proteins into smaller amino acids)
- Co-enzyme Q10 twice a day (This is an anti-oxidant which helps boost energy levels)
- Hawthorn capsules twice a day (to protect the heart and slow and steady the heartbeat.)
- Magnesium Orotate – twice a day (This form of magnesium is easily absorbed and supports the heart.)

23rd June 2022 - 2nd online consultation.

Her headaches and fatigue were greatly improved. Chest heaviness was still a concern but had also improved. Overall she was extremely happy with such a big improvement in her health.

My Treatment

Continue -

- co-enzyme Q10,

- hawthorn
- magnesium orotate.

Add herb tonic with –

- 5 types of mushroom (for the immune system), arjuna (a heart tonic) and astragalus (to support the immune system and increase white blood cells)

21st July 2022 - 3rd online consultation.

She was feeling great, and back to her old self. I recommended that she take vitamin C, vitamin D and zinc to further support her immune system. I recommended that she re-test her blood after two months and contact me for another appointment should the bloods still show a low white blood cell count. I haven't heard anything from her so I assume this test must have been good.

Case Study 3: Healing after Pfizer and Moderna shots

My patient was a 59 year-old storeman. He cycled and walked regularly. He was slightly overweight but was in relatively good health.

He had the first Pfizer shot on 22nd July 2021 and the second Pfizer shot on 12th August 2021. He had no symptoms or reactions except that he felt a little tired after each one. The third shot was Moderna on 24th February 2022 and again, other than fatigue, he showed no particular symptoms. However, over the next few months the fatigue became worse and he started to get a persistent cough. At first it was just a little at night, then morning as well, accompanied by shortness of breath which was also getting worse. He went to the doctor and had x-rays and blood testing which showed mild emphysema, a mild lung infection and long covid - even though he couldn't remember ever having had covid.

Lymphocytes and eosinophils (both types of white blood cells) were three times as high as normal for him, which indicated a blood disorder leading to asthma and might even be associated with leukaemia.

The doctor prescribed antibiotics and an asthma inhaler - neither of which made him feel any better.

6th September 2022 - 1st online consultation.

He blamed his symptoms on the covid shots as he described feeling a little off after the first two and shrugging it off, until his health went into a definite decline after the third shot. He had never experienced any fatigue or lung issues before.

By this time, he had been feeling tired, weak and breathless for months and it was interfering with his day-to-day living. He was beginning to feel that he would never recover.

My Treatment

- Pfizer 200c homeopathic twice a week for 2 weeks
- Moderna 200c homeopathic twice a week for 2 weeks
- Mushroom complex 3 times a day to clear the lungs and balance the immune system
- Quercetin - 4 times a day (histamine response – to open airways)

- NAC - twice a day (for lung congestion and detoxing)
- Serrapeptase - 3 x day to dissolve unwanted proteins
- Herb tonic – 8 mls day – including mullein (antibacterial, anti-inflammatory which supports lung function) and adhatoda – an ayurvedic remedy for asthma and emphysema
- Zinc 50 mg day

27th September 2022 - 2nd online consultation. He was feeling a lot better. He was only coughing when the air was cold. His fatigue had improved, but he was by no means back to his former self. He was still suffering with shortness of breath and had developed some persistent low-grade headaches.

My Treatment

We continued the treatment. When the Moderna 200c was finished, we changed to

- Arsenicum album 30c homoepathic for the shortness of breath.

And added

- Zinc: 50mg per day. (This boosts the immune

system and allows the cells to absorb nutrients more easily.)

- Increased water consumption, and lots of live high water-content foods like grapes, watermelon, celery and cucumber for hydration, detoxing and preventing headaches.

14th November 2022 - 3rd consultation.

His fatigue had improved greatly. His shortness of breath had stayed the same but his cough suddenly escalated again. He felt he may have picked up a cold or a virus as he had a fever for a few nights. He had another X-ray and blood tests with everything coming back clear. He was told to increase his use of the asthma inhaler.

My Treatment

Continue as before. Plus:

- Lung herbs: Inulin, licorice and baptisia

22nd December 2022 - 4th consultation.

He was feeling much improved and more like himself again. His lungs were not yet 100% and he had a lingering cough but he was feeling pretty good .

My Treatment

Continue herbal tonic

- NAC once a day
- Mushroom complex once a day
- Zinc once a day
- Vitamin C 500mg - 3x per day
- Vitamin D 5000iu per day for 2 months

He contacted me via text to cancel his next appointment. The combination of the protocols and time off over Christmas meant that he was feeling back to his old self again. He wasn't taking any pharmaceutical medication. We agreed that he would call me if his health started to go downhill again and this hasn't happened.

He thanked me profusely for really listening to him describe the issues he was facing and prescribing only what was necessary to his recovery.

Rebel Tucker

A qualified Naturopath and Yoga Therapist with over 30 years' experience, Rebel encourages her clients to create well-being with traditional practices and yoga.

htps://www.yogarebel.com.au

Our covid experience

As a naturopath, I've seen clients both in person and online who have reported feeling unwell since having the covid vaccines. Some clients took these vaccines willingly and now regret their choice. Most felt that they had been forced to take the shots against their wishes.

Some have had mild symptoms that resolved quickly. Others have had more serious complications that their medical professionals could neither explain nor offer advice about. Some have seen medical professionals who actually admitted that their symptoms were due to the vaccines yet were able to offer them no help.

It's encouraging to hear of some doctors and specialists reacting sympathetically to clients and admitting that they have been vaccine injured.

Some clients had fallen sick with one or more bouts of covid *after* the vaccines. All of them sensed that they had reacted to the vaccines rather than fallen prey to the illness itself. Most of the medical tests they had undergone were inconclusive or negative, and, despite their symptoms, many of these clients were not given any advice. Many had even been dismissed by their medical professionals as being overly reactive to scaremongering.

A little closer to home; an elderly family member collapsed within days of the covid vaccine and was taken to hospital. Despite the correlation they refused to entertain that it might have been due to the vaccine. Another family member ended up in intensive care for five days just 24 hours after their second covid vaccine.

As owners of a small health food store, my husband and I hear stories of harm and loss from our clients that can only link back to the covid vaccines. Some of these people report personal harm such as confirmed cardiomyopathy, pericarditis, headaches, and body pain. Most of them now realise that the decline in their health was due to the shots.

When they speak of their family members or friends, they tell accounts of sudden death, turbo cancers, heart disease, chronic pain and fatigue, paralysis, POTS, (postural orthostatic tachycardia syndrome, or disturbingly irregular heart rate and blood pressure) vertigo, dizziness, and declined cognitive function. Many tell us that friends and family are either in denial that the vaccines had anything to do with their health concerns or that they are now living with regret that they ever complied. They question the integrity of the medical establishment because of the harm done to them that they can only attribute to the vaccines.

It's sad that so many have been dismissed with the well-worn phrase, *'it's just in your head'* by their medical professionals, and it is encouraging that some have had more sympathetic reactions. Of course, these testimonies are 'only stories', they are 'just anecdotal', but I'm inclined to believe these people because of the level of conviction of these personal accounts and because nothing else explains their symptoms. Here are a few case reports.

As usual, when I saw these clients in my clinic, I took a thorough case history and, based on symptoms, applied the best-fit naturopathic medicines with varying rates of success. *Most of them had already self-prescribed a wide range of supplements based on their own research*. Most had applied a common covid treatment protocol and some had applied a protocol for adverse reactions to the covid vaccines.

Case Study 1: Recovery from 2 Pfizer shots

A 44-year-old stay at home mum with three young children. She was generally fit and well. She decided to take the shots as she felt pressured by other people. After having the vaccines, she had experienced persistent lethargy and shortness of breath She then contracted covid *twice* and the shortness of breath grew worse. Her symptoms had been ongoing for about 6 months. She had gone to the doctor and been referred for all sorts of tests which she had not done yet. Her shortness of breath was obvious but when I measured the oxygen levels of her blood, they were normal. She felt stressed and anxious and was feeling as if this breathing difficulty would never go away. She had resolved never to get any further covid shots as her own experience, plus stories she was hearing from friends, had alerted her to possible problems.

Symptoms:

- Lethargy after the 1st vaccine, plus shortness of breath after the 2nd vaccine
- She became sick with covid for the first time:
- She had two months of coughing

She had self-prescribed:

- Zinc
- Quercetin
- Vitamin C
- Vitamin D3
- Melatonin

She had covid a *second* time a few months later with the same symptoms. This time the shortness of breath was worse. The doctor had prescribed an asthma inhaler and she continued the same sort of supplement protocol she had taken for the first bout of covid.

My Treatment:

- Practitioner Product: 9500 IU Vitamin A, Papain, Amylase, 380 IU Vitamin D3
- Nattokinase: 125mg twice a day
- N-Acetyl Cysteine – 1g twice a day. (This supports the production of the body's most important antioxidants to support the immune system and helps with elimination of toxins.)
- Herbal Mix: Echinacea, Elderflower, Eyebright, Thyme, and Liquorice 5 ml three times a day
- Lung - meridian – I suggested backbends and heart opening practices to stimulate the lungs and chest area.
- Yogic Breathing Practices: Alternate Nostril breathing (Nadi Shodhana) support lowering of stress, blood pressure and improved concentration.

Progression:

2nd Treatment - 1 month later: Symptoms were improved but not completely gone

- I added Ubiquinol 300mg per day. (This is a form of Co-enzyme Q-10 which is more readily usable by the body to provide more energy to the cells, help your organs perform better and protect cells from oxidation)
- I encouraged her to do the breathing practice more regularly

Results:

Approximately 6 weeks later:

- The shortness of breath had resolved, and fatigue had really improved
- We agreed that she should finish all other supplements and stay on the Ubiquinol for another month.
- She resolved to be proactive and look after her health and that of her family with healthy eating and lifestyle habits.

Case Study 2: Healing after being coerced into taking a shot

A 52-year-old female aged-care manager and administrator. She didn't want to take the shot. After much thought and effort to maintain her work *without* the covid vaccines, she finally caved-in to keep her job and took it against her wishes. She felt tired and lethargic afterwards, and a few days later developed back and neck pain and a severe headache. She was hot and felt 'as if her head was going to explode'. She went to the Emergency Department in hospital where blood tests and scans ruled out blood clots. She was told it was all in her mind. She was very emotional, disappointed in herself for having the vaccine and angry at being forced into it to keep her job.

She had been taking a protocol of Zinc, Vitamin C, Vitamin D3, Ubiquinol and Fish Oil.

Symptoms:

- Persistent back and neck pain
- Severe headache
- Fatigue
- Anxiety and emotional distress

My Treatment:

- Reiki (energy healing)
- Increased Vitamin D3 to 5000IU per day
- Added N-acetyl cysteine to 200mg x 3 times a day
- Increased Ubiquinol to 300mg per day
- Added Vit E Complex 120mg twice per day

Mindfulness practice:

- Acceptance
- Breathing – deep inhales, hold and long exhales.

Results:

10 days later she was feeling much better and felt as if she had turned a corner. The breathing practices really helped to calm her down.

Her headache had resolved.

- She decided to more spiritual practices as well as psychology.
- She had resolved to have no further covid vaccines.

Case Study 3: A business owner recovers

A 47-year-old man who runs his own businesses. He was busy and fit, with no prior health concerns. He had his first covid vaccine and was immediately unwell with dizziness, fatigue, and vertigo triggered by bright lights so bad that he would end up on the ground. His ability to run his businesses came to a standstill and his wife had to take over many of the responsibilities. He had a barrage of tests done, including brain scans, and was told by the doctor that he believed his symptoms were an adverse reaction to the covid vaccine. *He had no solutions for him* and he was told to manage his stress. He had already tried vitamin C, Vitamin D3, Zinc, Quercetin and N-Acetyl Cystiene but his symptoms were persistent and unrelenting. These had been ongoing for almost nine months.

Symptoms:

- Dizziness – diagnosed by GP as POTS (postural orthostatic tachycardia syndrome, or disturbingly irregular heart rate and blood pressure)

- Chronic and unrelenting fatigue.
- Mental fog
- Pain in his arms and legs
- Shortness of breath

My Treatment:

- Nattokinase: 125mg twice a day
- Ubiquinol: 300mg twice a day for 2 months

Results:

After 4 weeks he reported that his symptoms had improved but were not completely gone. He was able to increase his ability to work, but still not to his full capacity

Progression:

- Reduced the dose of Ubiquinol to 300mg once a day
- Maintained the dose of Nattokinase for another month

Results:

This patient didn't return for another consultation, but reported that he felt he had moved in the right direction and was well on his way to feeling completely well. He attributes his health decline to the covid vaccines and will never have another.

Anonymous

(For entertainment purposes only. Chlorine dioxide is a water purifier.)

Case Study 1: Healing with Chlorine Dioxide (MMS)

Late in 2021 a 26 year-old woman with no underlying health issues became ill with what was thought to be Covid 19. Although she didn't take a test her symptoms were in line with a severe flu with many of the covid symptoms. It started with her throat becoming very inflamed to the point she was finding it hard to swallow. As the days went on she became very tired and her breathing was laboured. She had full body aches and headaches with fever and chills.

By the time she contacted me for help she was already 5 days into it and was very sick.

She couldn't get out of bed for very long and she had to wear an eye patch over her eyes as the light was too strong for her to bear.

I started her off on nutraceuticals which included high dose vitamin c, d, zinc and quercetin. She also had some ivermectin that she had taken on day 5. As she started this treatment quite late into her illness it didn't have any effect. Nothing seemed to be helping and her symptoms were getting worse.

I told her that she really needed to go to hospital but she refused. She didn't want to be put on the hospital protocols of Remdesivir (which was causing kidney failure) and ventilation which seemed to be making people worse. As the days passed, she continued to decline and started to get severe sharp pains in her chest area which indicated pneumonia or sepsis. She still refused to go to the hospital.

Three months before this I had seen some information about a product called MMS (Miracle Mineral Solution or Chlorine Dioxide) I personally had never heard of this product but discovered that it had been used successfully for many years as a water purifying agent. There were also claims about its miraculous healing properties, including healing Covid 19. I didn't really believe these claims but I had ordered some of the product, mainly for water purifying, and put it in the cupboard.

The patient was now day 10 into her illness and still refusing to go to the hospital, I was very worried and concerned for her life. I had run out of the 'usual' things to try when I suddenly remembered I had the Miracle Mineral Solution product sitting in my cupboard.

As I had nothing to lose, I started her on a low dose. As she handled that well I increased the dose throughout the day and by the evening, she got out of bed for the first time without her eye patch, and was well enough to eat.

In the following days she continued to get better and by the end of the third day of taking MMS she had made full recovery with no lingering symptoms at all.

As I saw this miraculous recovery right before my very eyes, I went on to research the healing power of Chlorine Dioxide more thoroughly and have come to understand why it has been suppressed by the pharmaceutical industry.

Case Study 2: Healing with Chlorine Dioxide (MMS)

A 48 year-old woman in good health with no underlying conditions took two Pfizer vaccines a few weeks apart. She had a mild reaction and a sore arm, but everything seemed to be fine.

About 3 months after the vaccinations her health started to deteriorate with many ongoing symptoms that saw her visiting the doctor on a weekly basis. She got 'covid' three times and her immune system was struggling to cope. Her symptoms included chronic fatigue, brain fog, numbness in her legs and what felt like electric shocks going through different parts of her body. Her muscles did not seem to be working well. She had severe gut issues and was constantly vomiting up whatever she tried to eat. As a consequence she lost a large amount of weight very quickly.

Her doctor could not work out what was going on so she was referred to a neurologist who ran all sorts of tests but could not find anything wrong. As time went on, she got a little better until she contracted 'covid' again for the fourth time and ended up in hospital as she was struggling to breathe and needed oxygen support. She was stabilized in hospital but when she came home she was in a severely depleted state and very weak.

I began to build her body back up with a range of vitamins, minerals and herbs as well as some probiotics to help with her gut issues.

She started to feel a little better but was still so chronically fatigued that any time she exerted herself slightly she would have to recover by sleeping for hours afterwards. To detox her body and to clear her of the toxic spike protein I put her on Chlorine Dioxide in the form of CDS. She started on a very low dose and gradually built up the number of drops over the next week. Within 2 weeks she reported that her symptoms were subsiding and she was getting her energy back. After four weeks of taking CDS on a daily basis she reported that she was back to the energy levels she had before she took the shots and all her symptoms resolved.

She is still doing well.

Spiritual aspects of Wellness

Emotional toxicity, programmed beliefs and baggage may hold you back from the healing you deserve. **Dr Bruce Lipton** describes how this works in his his book **The Biology of Belief**. If you are serious about healing yourself from long covid or an injection injury you may need to let go of a swag of negative emotions thoughts and beliefs. You may need to forgive yourself. You may even need to let go of some of the negative people in your life. You'll know who they are by the way you feel when you're around them or the relief you feel after they leave. There are many courses that can help with this but ultimately it is your journey.

You may find it helpful to buy a special book and write down in detail the painful things in your life that need to be released.

As you are writing, understand your part in all this, and let it go anyway, spilling any frustration, pain or grief onto the page. Writing these things down means that you don't need to carry them around in your head or your heart any more. You might like to write a few main points on a piece of paper and perform a ritual of throwing them onto the fire or ripping them up into tiny pieces but if you should ever need this information for any reason, you can dig out the book again.

Visualise being well in great detail. The body is an amazing and miraculous instrument and you're still here. Remember that we are all, in essence, energy. If scientists peer into the contents of a single atom, there is nothing there but a few tiny particles and a lot of space. **Amazingly, those particles can actually be seen responding to the attention they are being given in any moment.**

A Japanese scientist called **Dr Masaru Emoto** added further proof of this when he conducted some amazing experiments with water in the 1990s and beyond. In his book, **'The Hidden Messages in Water'**, he photographed ice crystals and found that those from water bathed in beautiful classical music or loving words were exquisite ice crystals. Those which were exposed to hateful words or insults had only lumpy and misshapen crystals. The results were the same in any language.

It is clear that the atoms and molecules of our body actually respond to our heart-felt words.

Few people describe this better than **Dr Joe Dispenza** in his book **'You are the Placebo'** in which he describes healing himself after a terrible road accident within weeks. He has taught these techniques ever since.

You can take heart from this story. Know that we are powerful creators and that anything is possible.

This is almost a story for our time as we contemplate the world today.

There is a chance that the covid era has impacted your life in ways you never thought possible. Your health, your family, your job, your sense of security and even your home may have been placed in the balance. I and my colleagues have done our best here in this little book to gather a few reliable resources to help you survive and thrive through this and I encourage you to take action to help yourself.

Service to others

There is also another side to this. The world is full of people who have been taken down to the depths of despair in a crisis situation of some sort and survived. It could have been the early death of a parent, It could have been an accident, an illness, a divorce, financial ruin, a near death experience or the death of a child. Nobody wants these things, but the crisis changed something in these people. It made them rethink their lives and in the following years they devoted themselves to helping others in similar situations.

Joe Dispenza is one of these: **Louise Hay** and **Chris Wark** cured themselves of cancer, **Wayne Dyer** spent his childhood in a series of foster homes; **Tony Robbins**' childhood with a series of step dads wasn't much better; **Ty and Charlene Bollinger** lost family members to cancer; **Polly Tommey, Mark Blaxill, Brian Hooker** and **J B Handley** have vaccine-damaged children in their twenties. **Robert F Kennedy Jr** famously lost both his uncle and his father in tragic circumstances.

What they went through and survived has driven them to seek out powerful ways of helping others for much of their lives

How will the covid era influence your life into the future...?

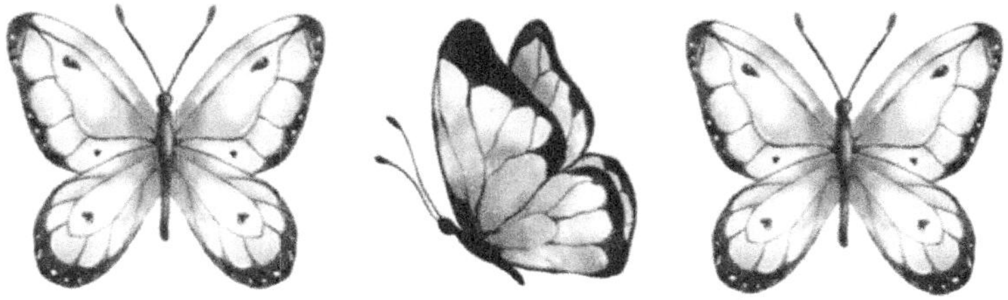

My wish for mankind is that we emerge from these
times with more clarity:
about who we really are...
about who we can really trust...
about how miraculous our bodies really are...
about how magnificent our planet really is...
and about how we take care of the things we value…
so we can all thrive together…

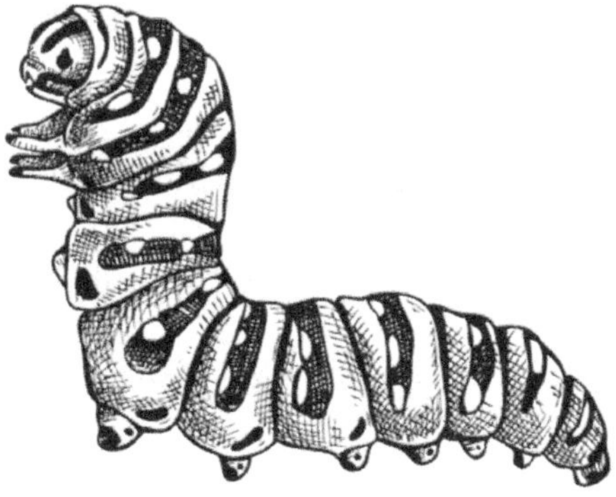

References and Links

The links and references are provided for further information which may be useful for a wide range of readers. Thousands of people around the world are dedicated to piecing this information together to help you.

If you are recovering, much of this information may not be for you at this stage and I encourage you to stay as uplifting, light, happy and optimistic as you can manage. In your reading, thoughts, emotions and habits.

Your 30 trillion cells are listening ….

As I checked and rechecked the links for this book, I learned to check for pesky gaps if I couldn't get the links to work

Vaccines, Myths and Facts:

An overview of the vaccine story, clear and simple, with big text, lots of pictures and over 100 references and links – available from:

https://www.inhousepublishing.com.au/

vaccines.light.of.truth@gmail.com

See links under 'Resource' on

https://www.lightoftruths.net/

Wendy Daniel talks about the 4th edition of 'Vaccines, Myths and Facts'

https://youtu.be/SfS03lYAZIQ?si=Ai3tJrljaHTroT_J.

A slightly longer talk:

https://youtu.be/
TgJOYKgNXRs?si=JrD0ruWc1k5QuCH4

Journal of Translational Science Health effects in vaccinated versus unvaccinated children, with covariates for breastfeeding status and type of birth. Brian Hooker, Neil Z Miller

Published: June 2021. Pubmed Website:

https://pubmed.ncbi.nlm.nih.gov/

type in PMID number: 32537156

HighWire with Del Bigtree - Weekly Rumble Show.

This is a massive resource covering the whole vaccine narrative. This type of information is heavily censored from mainstream media and all the major channels including YouTube and Facebook. In today's world it only proves its validity.

Books

Book: The Juice Lady's Guide to Juicing for Health - Cherie Calbom

Book: The War on Ivermectin - Dr Pierre Kory

The Medicine that saved Millions and could have ended the Pandemic. A book by Dr Pierre Kory, a founding member of the FLCCC

Book: There is a cure for Diabetes - Dr Gabriel Cousens

Dr Cousens would be in his eighties by now but a few years ago I spent three weeks at his retreat in Arizona, and saw this program in action. I was impressed with the amount of time he spent with us, sharing his profound wisdom and insight.

Book: You are the Placebo. Dr Joe Dispenza

He has a huge amount of knowledge on his website and does regular healing and visualization retreats.

https://drjoedispenza.com/

Book: The Biology of Belief - Bruce Lipton PhD

Book: The Wisdom of Your Cells - Bruce Lipton PhD

Bruce Lipton speaks powerfully about how our thoughts influence the performance of our miraculous cells

https://youtu.be/WSW2MszpK-0?si=1tP5kw9PDbR3LLVe

Book: You can Heal Your Life - Louise Hay

Book: The Cure for all Diseases - Hulda Regehr Clark

Book: The Cure for all Advanced Cancers - Hulda Regehr Clark.

(and several more, available on Amazon)

General Health Videos

Dr Eric Berg - has a huge library of simple, concise natural health information on YouTube.

Dr Mark Hyman - has a wealth of longer natural health videos and interviews with many health researchers on YouTube.

Barbara O'Neill - In more enlightened times Barbara O'Neill might be respected as a wise woman with a wealth of knowledge, common sense and hands on experience. These qualities are not always welcomed by the medical industry. I invite you to seek out her talks on YouTube and draw your own conclusions. You'll recognise her by her calm, steady voice and large whiteboard. Facebook posts using her name are probably imitations.

Chris Wark – Chris Beat Cancer, the Square One program.

https://www.chrisbeatcancer.com/

https://squareone.chrisbeatcancer.com/login

5 Amazing benefits of Grass Fed Butter: Dr Eric Berg

https://youtu.be/JttjTjKEpuc?si=RIwHC_LiYIxleaen

Dr Eric Berg speaks about the advantages of eating eggs

https://youtu.be/--Rx7EZyC7s?si=qx6CSTM-VGG2V94T

Ben Carpenter talks about how they fatten up lab rats:

https://youtu.be/Jhu7_Fo_qF8?si=dSYRrabSXRgMsO25

No wonder we all put on weight so easily!

Chris Van Tulleken talks about ultra-processed foods

https://youtu.be/5QOTBreQalk?si=Ig3kZnPrCW07ebmL

The Vladimir Zelenko protocols

https://vladimirzelenkomd.com/treatment-protocol/

https://zstacklife.com/pages/about-dr-vladimir-zelenko-md

Bakersfield Doctors speak about what they were seeing on April 20 2020

https://www.turnto23.com/news/coronavirus/watch-controversial-press-conference-held-by-two-bakersfield-doctors-that-was-pulled-down-by-youtube

Dr John Campbell talks about excess death rates in 2023.

https://youtu.be/_6xBiyidQ9g?si=5-wi7cEc8DmGSSyY

This is just one of many regular talks which Dr John Cambell has presented. Initially pro-covid vaccine, he *followed the evidence wherever it led* and, like so many others, is shocked by what he has seen unfold.

The World Council for Health

https://worldcouncilforhealth.org/resources/a-practical-approach-to-keeping-healthy-after-your-covid-19-jab/--

https://worldcouncilforhealth.org/resources/spike-protein-detox-guide/

World of Wellness

https://wowintl.org/#

The Front Line Covid 19 Critical Care Alliance (FLCCC Alliance)

https://covid19criticalcare.com/

The Wellness Company

https://www.twc.health/

Dr Phillip Altman talks to former president of the AVN, Meryl Dorey.

https://rumble.com/v33bf7y-under-the-wire-a-conversation-with-dr-phillip-altman-covid-jabs-and-myocard.html

Dr Peter McCullough, a cardiologist speaks about the demonisation of tried-and-true early treatments

https://fb.watch/o6lvHaLObm/?mibextid=v7YzmG

Dr Peter McCullough is on the Substack platform app under *Courageous Discourse* and speaks out consistently, citing the latest robust research papers and government statistics.

Colonic Hydrotherapy/ colonic irrigation

https://www.naturaltherapypages.com.au/natural_medicine/colon_irrigation

Michael Gray Griffith from Café Locked out speaks with Craig Kelly, who is now with the One Nation party

https://rumble.com/v3tmpt8-a-slow-chat-with-craig-kelly.-a-cafe-locked-out-interview.html

Chlorine Dioxide, the Universal Antidote lost documentaries series

https://theuniversalantidote.com/the-universal-antidote-lostdocumentaries-series/

(for entertainment purposes only)

Spooky 2

https://www.spooky2.com

Check out the Generator X Pro essential kit for accurate biofeedback or start off with the more modest Spooky 2 portable essential kit if budget is a consideration. You will need a Windows computer to load the programs.

Dr. Thomas Lodi Parasites Webinar

https://drlodi.com/

Has a webinar on the cancer/parasite link and lists detailed anti-parasitic protocols (behind a modest paywall).

Dr Thomas Lodi and Dr Edward Group talk about parasites and cancer

https://youtu.be/0Sxu8iGnOCA?si=zLqSeDcyHtXlPZvf

Dr Bryan Ardis

https://thedrardisshow.com

Dr Bryan Ardis has regular interviews with many well known and trusted professionals and has a range of supplements available on his website:

The Medical Rebel

https://www.drleemerritt.com/

Dr Lee Merritt, has some great interviews and healing protocols on her website

Dr Janine Bowring ND speaks about parasite and candida remedies

https://youtu.be/LfrnMA5VSVQ?si=42M9t-yECEpmglQ4

Dr Eric Berg talks about signs you have parasites
https://youtu.be/P2dLjZxGAc4?si=_lApZLV4OaUtGh1T

plus others on parasites

Eric Berg talks about Nattokinase and its powerful anti clotting effects
https://youtu.be/Cf6ux-mRP2k?si=lWifld25zfczD4mL

Oncologist Dr Makis speaks with Jim Ferguson about covid and turbo cancers in October 2023
https://rumble.com/v3ssk1q-must-watch-dr.-william-makis-on-turbo-cancer-ive-never-seen-cancers-behavin.html

Gynaecologist Dr James Thorp and a nurse whistleblower talk about the rise in foetal deaths following the covid shots.
https://rumble.com/v1ugjo4-whistleblower-nurse-exposes-rise-in-fetal-demise.html

Jefferey Jaxen talks about maternal mortality after the covid shots on the HighWire
https://rumble.com/v49hzhl-is-a-spike-in-maternal-mortality-connected-to-the-cdc.html

Dr. Paul Marik on The Covid-19 Vaccine vs Natural Infection.

https://rumble.com/v2t89rw-outstanding-interview-with-dr.-paul-marik-includes-exceptional-health-heali.html

American Thought Leaders

theepochtimes.com/epochtv/american-thought-leaders

The Epoch Times has some great interviews with health professionals @AmericanThoughtLeaders

One answer to Cancer

https://youtu.be/eyPSHzJDEqo?si=DAZ3VC2BhpPvv-rh

No description of censored cancer treatments is complete without Elaine Hollingsworth's documentary on Black Salve: One answer to Cancer

Oncologist William Makis MD reviews 9 research papers on the treatment of cancers with Ivermectin:

https://open.substack.com/pub/makismd/p/ivermectin-and-cancer-it-has-at-least?r=149bj4&utm_medium=ios&utm_campaign=post

The **Substack** app is quite a learned and serious platform where you will find in depth health topics. If you are a non-medically qualified person recovering from toxicity of any form I don't recommend wading into these discussions.

Remember that your body hears your thoughts, words and emotions and it pays to keep them light and optimistic when in recovery mode.

These are posted as a few more starter points and possible clues for those seeking more answers for you.

Courageous Discourse: Dr Peter McCullough:
World renowned Heart specialist

COVID Intel: Dr William Makis:
Canadian oncologist

Philip Altman's Substack:
former Australian pharmaceutical regulator

Pierre Kory's Medical Musings: The War on Ivermectin:
US doctor and author:

Humanity United Now: Dr Ana Maria Mihalcea:
Ana is an EDTA specialist in the US and has written consistently about the possibility of nano technology in covid vaccines.

The political football

If you are recovering, you may also not feel strong enough to listen to ethical Australian sites covering Covid as a political football, including:

Club Grubbery, with Graham Hood and John Larter (Facebook)

Interviews and discussions about what is happening in Australia

Café Locked Out with Michael Gray Griffith (Facebook)

Interviews from around the country

The Forest of the Fallen

https://theforestofthefallen.com/

Occasional memorials to the Australian injured which you might see fluttering in the breeze in your local park or headland.

Get ahead of Cancer: Education and Empowerment.

Candace Bradstreet is a Certified Clinical Nutritionist and Health Coach who worked for some years with her brother-in-law, the late Jeff Bradstreet, who many of us knew as one of the top autism doctors in the world.

She has a small and interesting range of supplements and treatments, including a Rife machine.

Facebook page: **Get ahead of Cancer: Education and Empowerment.**

https://ourlittlewhitebarn.com/

What does a chiropractor actually do?

https://youtu.be/yTIO79KFVuE?si=YmY4PHd9ciZVOYZ-

Class Action Lawsuits

Class Action lawsuits are those where lawyers represent dozens or hundreds of people with similar grievances, often choosing a couple of examples of harm to represent everyone. At the same time as you are empowering yourself to heal, look out for these in your country if you have had an injury or suffered financial harm. Track down the date and batch number of the jabs you were given, Note your symptoms and the dates, times and interactions with your doctor. Don't hold your breath, but you may be eligible for compensation.

Dr William Bay (Suspended for speaking out against the covid shots) interviews Dr Melissa McCann about the class action lawsuit for people damaged physically or financially by the Covid injections.

https://fb.watch/phCYfyksc9/?mibextid=v7YzmG

https://www.covidvaxclassaction.com.au/

Dr Melissa McCann, a brave advocate for patients in Australia, talks here to Dr John Campbell.

https://youtu.be/UIF2omTmFVM?si=Gu469V8vw5kyklhF

https://www.sydneycriminallawyers.com.au/blog/class-action-commenced-over-covid-19-vaccine-injuries/

March 2024: United Australia Party (UAP) Senator Ralph Babet finally managed to put through a Bill in The Australian Senate to launch a world-first formal inquiry.

https://dailydeclaration.org.au/2024/03/27/australian-senate-launches-world-first-formal-inquiry-into-excess-mortality/

Asenatecommitteehasbeentaskedwithinvestigating the reasons for Australia's highest excess mortality rates since World War 2, with a report due in August 2024

TGA: Theraputic Goods Administration:

Which is supposed to regulate therapeutic goods like medicines and vaccines.

AHPRA: The Australian Health Practitioner Regulation Agency.

Naturopaths:

Lee Clarke: The Body of Natural Health
https://www.thebodyofnaturalhealth.com.au

Patricia Vandenberg-Smith: Journey to Health
https://journeytohealth.com.au

Rebel Tucker
http://yogarebel.com.au

Suppliers:

My Health Food Shop
https://myhealthfoodshop.com.au/

This online store has a physical store in Castle Hill, Western Sydney and offers a vast range of supplements and other health products. I encourage you to support your local health stores if you have them, but this range is impressive.

Wellness kits (in Australia)

https://www.thebodyofnaturalhealth.com.au/product-page/immunity-pack

Miracle Products

This is a Queensland supplement brand I have been familiar with for some years. I have always appreciated their high-quality formulations I have come to depend on for my own fitness.

When I asked one of the partners what they would select as a response to covid, methylene blue (Blu-Zone) was the first response for those who hadn't taken the shots. (It's very blue. Don't spill it on your kitchen bench!)

It's a powerful support for the cells, clearing toxins and parasites.

Other support products include Vitamin C, Zinc, C60, Camu Camu, Life Force electrolyte formula and Activated Gold Curcumin.

Their stabilised CDS food grade water purifier tabs are a good choice for clearing pathogens (disease producing nasties) from water and blood.

The website includes many interesting articles *https://miracleproducts.shop/*

Iherb

https://au.iherb.com/

Dr Bryan Ardis has a range of supplements

https://thedrardisshow.com/

Global Healing: Naturopath Dr Edward Group

I caught Dr Ed Group talking on a discussion panel about checking the quality of supplements and how they can be compromised.

Discernment is key but his words gave me confidence in products from this company.

https://globalhealing.com/

DAEN

(Database of Adverse Event Notifications) is the Australian TGA (Theraputic Goods Administration) website for reporting adverse reactions from medicines including vaccines of all types. It is not easy to interpret the data in there.

If you have had ad adverse event following a covid shot I encourage you to report it. Your doctor should have the record of the batch number of your shot on his files.

OpenDAEN.Info is a site created entirely by volunteers and launched in January 2024 which sorts the DAEN data on the covid shots (initially) into an understandable format which can be easily read and interpreted by public and professionals alike. They have also incorporated Australian Batch numbers and linked them with numbers of adverse reactions. *https://opendaen.info*

Made in the USA
Monee, IL
04 November 2026

67381730R10098